I BLAME THE HORMONES

LIVING WITH REPRODUCTIVE DEPRESSION

I BLAME THE HORMONES

LIVING WITH REPRODUCTIVE DEPRESSION

CAROLINE CHURCH

First published by Harper Collins as a HarperTrue Short Read in 2015
This revised and fully expanded edition published by Albert Bridge Books 2021

DISCLAIMER

I am not a doctor or in any way a medical professional. Nothing I have written here should be considered medical advice and there are some elements to my testimony that others may find triggering.

The hormonal illnesses that I've described in this book, and which can manifest from the onset of puberty until the menopause, can be experienced by women and those who were assigned female at birth. I have used inclusive language wherever possible.

TABLE OF CONTENTS

FOREWORD

Caroline Church has produced a fascinating account of her journey from adolescence with depression and anxiety. Her testimony could be a best seller if it was expanded into a novel but as it is it's a very important document on the problems faced by women everywhere. It is a compelling and constructive account with great clarity, lacking in self-pity.

As she says in the title, she blames her hormones for her disturbances and she is correct. There is a transition in her story from painful periods to severe premenstrual depression followed by post-natal depression. She notes that she was very well during pregnancy, was better breast-feeding with the new baby but any new and abrupt hormonal changes bought about a recurrence of severe depression. Oestrogens helped but she had problems with the progestin components of hormonal therapy which led to a hysterectomy at the age of forty-two.

In her account she has perfectly described reproductive depression, which is a hormonal-based depression in women of reproductive age. This syndrome relates to the progress from premenstrual depression, post-natal depression and menopausal depression, noting that these depressive symptoms disappear during pregnancy.

The schematic description of her progress noted in the timeline of events at the start of the self-help section should be in textbooks of psychiatry because unfortunately psychiatrists have little knowledge of the concept of hormone-related depression and its effective treatments. Gynaecologists know that this problem can be helped or even cured by oestrogens but is often made worse by the progestin-containing forms of birth control. It also does not respond well to repeated courses of antidepressants.

Caroline's title *I Blame the Hormones* says it all. We must all learn from her compelling story.

Professor John Studd is founder of the London PMS and Menopause Clinic, and President of the National Osteopathic Society. He is also chairman of the British Menopause Society.

INTRODUCTION

This testimony is dedicated to the thousands of women worldwide who have yet to understand the direct relationship between their poor mental health and hormonal timing. I hope it will also educate the health care professionals who are unfamiliar with this coherent strategy which is proven to work.

Many times I have questioned why such an unfathomable disorder came to be part of me. I've looked at my genetic profile, environmental issues and family dynamics. I've questioned psychiatrists, endocrinologists and have even been hypnotized to see if I can uncover the fundamental reasons as to why I've been so unwell.

Unfortunately for many of us with the same disorder there isn't yet an answer. We have grown to accept our fate and life is unpredictable for all of us.

My endless searching for validation has been exhausting and often soul destroying. I can think of nothing good to come of living with a disease that causes acute misery and anguish. I do, however, have the utmost respect for the human body and all of its idiosyncrasies which are both miraculous and intriguing.

The reproductive system itself is so wondrous I can hardly find the words to convey the massive feat of endurance required by women who are making a baby. To be able to grow a small human being and then give birth has to be the most amazing accomplishment, even if at times it goes wrong. Quite often the physical elements to reproduction are flawed and can cause great hardship, as my own story shows.

I Blame the Hormones can help you to understand the correlation between your endocrine system and poor mental health. This then opens up a new vista of treatment options. It is also a relief to feel validated and understood in a world that is often dismissive of reproductive depression and all its manifestations.

The trajectory of this condition from puberty until menopause is long, and the emotional fallout incomprehensible. This disease doesn't discriminate and often creates enormous trauma for both the person concerned and their family. It destroys friendships and even has the ability to curtail successful careers. Don't, however, let my story put you off. There is great hope for the future for those that are suffering.

We are beginning to stigma-bust the notions that come with talking and treating mental illness, particularly when surrounding the menstrual cycle and childbearing years. One day, anyone who is suffering will be asked the simple question of whether they are in the late luteal phase of their cycle or whether their symptoms are cyclical. Women in their menopausal years will be taken more seriously when they say that they are suicidal or have multiple physical ailments. In the near future there will be more proven treatment plans and medical gas lighting will cease. This will undoubtedly improve the outlook for everyone who is suffering.

This alone has made me more determined to get my own story into circulation. I hope it will transform the lives of others and validate their suffering which is often overlooked within this field of medicine. Raising awareness is always paramount, as is the prevention of suicide.

Caroline Church, January 2021

PART 1

MEMOIR

PUBERTY – 1980S
THE TRANSITION INTO WOMANHOOD AND A PERSONALITY CHANGE

Growing up in the 1970s, I came from an ordinary working-class family and, although there was an underlying sense of financial difficulty, there was always food on the table and an abundance of love. As I started junior school there was no hint of the heartache to come, and I simply enjoyed life, being popular and surrounded by neighbours and friends I loved. I had a regular life, free of responsibility, with a mum who worked tirelessly in the home. My formative years were spent playing games and, during the summers, being out enjoying the long days. We would return when we were hungry and not before, when we would grab a snack and be on our way, without a care in the world.

When I was just ten years old, Mum told my younger sister and me that she had a surprise for us. We both waited patiently while she explained that she was going to have another baby, and even though this news was unexpected, we were both overjoyed and couldn't wait to be her willing helpers. I remember being fascinated and intrigued by her growing bump, and would often pretend to be Caroline the midwife with my stethoscope and nurse's case, while she allowed me to examine her tummy and listen for the sounds inside. Sometimes the baby would get the hiccups, which would make me squeal with delight. It was a joyful and happy time for us all as we waited for the baby to be born.

At the time, we lived in a large block of flats where there was a communal garden and the sense of a very close community. As children we would play the days away, happy and carefree. I was surrounded by little ones; often my baby sisters, and sometimes one of the neighbours would allow me to bath or feed their baby while they got on with their chores. I simply couldn't wait to have my own child, and I would often walk my sisters in their prams and pretend they were mine. People would stop to admire them and ask me about them, and I just felt so proud that they belonged to me and were so angelic to look at.

By the time I reached puberty, happiness gradually started to leave me; my struggle with depression had begun. I couldn't figure out why I had this sudden change in personality. I felt immediately different and very alone as I tried to make sense of what was happening to me. It seemed to come out of nowhere, and I remember feeling dreadfully insecure, intensely sad and sorrowful, though I couldn't say why. It was as if someone else had moved into my body and hijacked my mind, as my thoughts seemed so different to the innocent ones of the past. I tried desperately to cover my despair and sense of anguish with a tough exterior, as I didn't want anyone to know how I was really feeling or somehow think that I was strange or different in some way.

Fundamentally, as time went by, I just felt as though something was missing and that I didn't fit in somehow. As I developed and changed, this feeling of despondency increased and I began to suffer from health worries and anxiety. It was then that I noticed my thoughts were becoming obsessive and hostile, and I would sometimes be preoccupied with death and morbidity, which would leave me feeling extremely frightened and alone. I was perpetually worried that something bad was going to happen to my parents and my sisters, and I would be obsessed with trying to protect them while lying awake at night, filled with dread and unwanted thoughts. The more my body changed, the more I noticed an increasing mental chatter, with the same thoughts going over and over, as if on a loop, and I would struggle to slow them down. This, of course, left me emotionally drained and sometimes physically exhausted, and I hated this whole change in my persona which seemed to materialize overnight as my body began to change.

When I was fourteen I started my periods and, being at an all-girls school, the realization hit me quite early that not everybody was suffering the way I was. The pain was something I hadn't anticipated, and would often leave me hunched over and unable to straighten. In lessons I would flush hot with embarrassment as the teacher was often a man and he would know that it was the first day of my period. More often than not, I would have to go to the nurse's office as the cramps were too much to bear and I needed to go home. On my way to the sick room I would vomit violently, over and over, and as I clung on to the toilet to stop myself from fainting, tears would stream down my face and my eyes would burn. I would be crouching on the filthy toilet floor, desperately trying to catch my breath as the agony seared straight through my legs and into my pelvis, from where it would wrap around my back. Once the purging had done its job, I would go to the sick room and curl up in the foetal position before falling into a deep sleep, which seemed to be the only respite from the month-to-month misery that was to increase throughout my adolescence.

As time went by, my change in mood went from bad to worse, and I started to experience my first feelings of paranoia. I began to believe that I wasn't wanted at home so I decided to move out far too prematurely, on completion of my school exams. I moved in with friends first, but convinced myself that they didn't really like me, so I moved again, into a rented house where the people were relative strangers. This, of course, had a disastrous effect on my state of mind, and I went downhill rapidly as I became more and more isolated. I started to drink alcohol, which helped enormously with my racing thoughts, and I gradually began to self-medicate as depression and anxiety took over my life. I would pour myself a drink and swallow hard, waiting for the calmness to envelop me like a warm blanket as it crept through my veins. It greatly relieved the feelings of tension, and I thought that I had found the perfect solution to my problems. Unknowingly, this was the beginning of my self-harming, as I desperately sought out ways to find relief from the crippling and worsening anguish within.

At around seventeen years of age I started working as an auxiliary nurse in a home for the elderly, which involved extremely long hours and probably did little to help my worsening condition; I would often have to ring in sick as I struggled to cope. I had also started to have intermittent sobbing episodes, sporadic days when I would begin to cry and often still be crying several hours later, which of course left me utterly exhausted. I just couldn't fathom why I seemed to have these issues, why I sometimes would be weeping for days with a deep sense of bereavement for no particular reason. I also had a ghostly feeling around me, which seemed to be getting worse, and I would sometimes feel a sudden eeriness that would leave me suspicious of everything around me. Even my bedroom and the house in which I lived would become spookily unfamiliar, and I would suddenly be terrified. I just couldn't explain it, and because I felt so ashamed of my thoughts and feelings I didn't tell anyone, which of course increased my sense of isolation.

As time went by, my racing thought process became so troublesome that I began to see a psychiatrist in the hope that he could help me make sense of what I was experiencing. I had gone from being a playful, happy child to a damaged young woman within a couple of years, and I epitomized the phrase 'troubled teen'. As a direct result of my crippling low self-esteem I was also becoming more and more promiscuous, which did little for my reputation and self-respect. I was desperately trying to fill the void at any cost, even if it meant compromising my integrity. I hadn't had a disturbed childhood and, as far as I was aware, I didn't have any emotional baggage or hidden trauma, so I was concerned by this side to my character. The sex had started to become another addiction, along with my dependence on alcohol.

Once I started to divulge my feelings and worries to the psychiatrist, he became very concerned and asked to see me weekly. I had started to harbour thoughts of violence and suicide, but I was also experiencing the ghostly feeling (known as depersonalization) more and more often. I began to suffer from nightmares and would wake in the night with a great feeling of impending doom and terror, which would then start the sobbing again and prevent me from working. My paranoia increased too: I would wake suddenly and my heart would race in my chest; I felt sure that somebody was in the room with me. This, of course, was terrifying and would sometimes happen over consecutive nights, so for a whole week I would be frightened to go to bed because of what was awaiting me.

The psychiatrist and I decided together that I would try a mild antidepressant, in the hope that it would slow me down and help with my persistent feelings of paranoia. I would often feel the need to sleep during the day, and would sometimes still be there 17 hours later. As soon as the relentless chatter in my racing mind stopped, I would then stay in bed for hours at a time, utterly exhausted and unable to function. The situation was abysmal and had started to impact severely on my whole life, though I still couldn't tell anybody for fear of what they might think of me.

I genuinely felt that my colleagues perceived me as strange, and I often felt left out, self-conscious and plagued with self-doubt. As the months went by and the depression increased, I became increasingly perplexed by this sudden change in my character and the helplessness within.

I had been taking the antidepressants for some weeks when I had my first out-of-control experience, and it has haunted me to this day. There had been a conflict of some kind at home with my parents and I returned to my lodgings, where the crying began. The sadness engulfed me and, as I sat alone, I felt that the whole of mankind had died and left me on my own. I really felt the grief and loneliness that anyone would feel in that situation, along with the eeriness that had been around me before. All the room felt so odd and dreamlike, but without the protection that a dream could bring, and I cried pitifully and long into the night. I didn't want to stay any more with all of this desolation and sorrow, and it seemed as though my heart was broken but without a cause. I picked up the bottle of pills, emptied the tablets out, crushed some of them up and placed them on my tongue. They tasted so bitter and I immediately gagged, so the rest I just swallowed with some wine that I had in the cupboard for sedation purposes. I didn't want to die as such, I just wanted the feelings of misery to leave me and, as I gradually fell asleep, I allowed the tension to leave my body and the anxiety simply melted away.

Fortunately, the landlord found me just in time, and at the hospital I remember waking up as the nurse held me down while she fed a pipe down my throat. I struggled against her and retched violently as I tried desperately to pull the tube out of my own stomach. I could feel it dragging along my insides. My efforts, of course, made the nurse angry, and she shouted at me to stop while she tried again. I was annoyed, as being asleep had made me forget the feelings I had been experiencing; I was so disappointed to be awake again and to have to face it all. As I fought her off, I looked at the lights above my head and my body suddenly became floppy, without anything left to give. I fell into a deep sleep, which lasted three days, and when I finally woke up, I have never felt so embarrassed and ashamed, as the reality of what I had done suddenly hit me.

The week following my suicide attempt was an absolute nightmare. On my release from hospital I returned to see my psychiatrist, and between us we decided that I needed more intensive treatment. I was initially quite pleased to be going into a psychiatric ward, as I felt that at last I would get the help I needed and I could at least get a diagnosis. The reality, however, was extremely different, and although the doctors and nurses were kind, I was surrounded by schizophrenics and people with bipolar. Some were extremely ill and were withdrawing from alcohol and drug addictions, which was painful to see and extremely frightening. One particular lady I secretly named the 'pacer', as she wandered endlessly backwards and forwards while chatting away to herself. She seemed to be having her very own conversation and was even answering herself in a different voice, while her husband looked on despairingly. She seemed so normal in some ways and yet so damaged at the same time, and I desperately wanted to reach out to her and help her through it, which of course was futile as I was clearly in need of help myself.

The first couple of days, I sat on a window ledge and gazed over the green while silently crying. I remember feeling so upset that my world had come to this, which was exacerbated by what was going on around me. Sometimes the patients would freak out and the nurses would wrestle them to the floor before one of them administered an injection. The nights were absolutely awful, and I would often lie awake, rigid and scared, while some other poor soul whimpered long into the early hours of the morning. One particular day, I found a soiled item of underwear on my bed, which did nothing to help my increasing paranoia, as

I believed it was a deliberate attack on me and I was again being watched. It was a sorry place to be and I felt more and more disturbed while I was there, which of course hindered any chance of recovery. As the days went on I couldn't wait to get out of there and, in comparison to what was happening around me, I just felt I was in the wrong place and so very, very alone.

When it was visiting time I could see the pain and confusion in my parents' eyes – my poor mum looked so worried. I had done such a good job of hiding my depressive state that they had no real idea of how bad things were; they had possibly even thought it was a desperate attempt to gain attention. I had tried to shelter my mum from what was really going on as she had the girls to look after, and, anyway, it would mean that I had failed in my quest to be an independent woman, which I had so desperately wanted to be. What I should have done was to return home to the sanctity of my family, but instead I just moved further away from them, towards the internal struggle that would go on to dominate my younger years and had already begun to ruin my life.

Once I left the unit, still none the wiser and without a firm diagnosis, I moved house quite quickly, thinking that it would help with my increasing symptoms. I started wondering if my illness was a lifestyle problem, and I thought that if I could move, it would make things better and I would find a miraculous cure. However, the stress of the move only created further problems, and I started to spend more time at the doctors with various ailments, which were by now becoming physical as well as emotional. I was referred to another unit where I would receive help for my increasing alcohol dependency and health anxieties, as the doctors felt that that my various neuroses were all part of the same 'personality disorder'. Although the health professionals were blaming my issues on a psychiatric element, I felt sure that there was something physically wrong with me, but my hunch was dismissed and I even started to believe that I was becoming a hypochondriac, questioning whether I was indeed ill or if it was all part of my imagination.

Despite this, I was experiencing extreme lower back pain and severe restless legs, which I insisted were menstrual-related, and I had a number of exploratory operations in the hope that a cause could be found. I had period pains even when I had no period, and the vomiting and fainting were relentless, even though I had been prescribed the contraceptive pill to help me. I had sporadic episodes of shaking and had developed a tremor in my hand, which was exacerbated by the amount of alcohol I was drinking to calm my symptoms. Eventually, I was detoxed, in the hope that it would stop me feeling endlessly unwell both in body and mind. I seemed to be going round and round in circles, and was in therapy at every opportunity, trying to gain some control over my life.

As I approached my early twenties I started to experiment with cannabis, using recreational drugs to attempt to help rid my body of the acute tension which was with me day in, day out. I was still in therapy, but I was now on stronger antidepressants and sometimes tranquillizers as well, in the hope that they would save me from the negative feelings and internalized pain. If things were really bad I would use a mood stabilizer, and then I would use Ecstasy at the weekends too. At one point I was using so many different concoctions and potions, trying to find anything to help me, it's a wonder that I was able to function at all. If I was really wired and agitated I would use alcohol, drugs and even sex to decipher my feelings and help me cope with the day-to-day misery of what the doctors had convinced me was a general depressive illness, which didn't have a physical element at all.

The problem with using recreational drugs and smoking cannabis was that they worked extremely effectively at controlling the feelings of tension, so by the time I was in my early twenties, my life had spiralled out of control. I was regularly feeling suicidal and permanently manic, and I was starting to experience delusions and wild imaginings, often believing that there was somebody living in my apartment with me. I would rush wildly around and then crash, sometimes for days at a time, while feelings of imminent doom and terror would wake me from the deepest sleep. I had a panic disorder which would cause me to imagine someone was following me, and I was on the edge of despair most days, believing that there was something living under my bed waiting to grab me. Sometimes I thought it had moved into my airing cupboard, and I would move past as quickly as possible in case it jumped out to get me! I was so filled with adrenalin I would run from task to task, even in my own flat, and I would imagine endless scenarios over and over again. I still had a preoccupation with death and would manage to convince myself that I was dying, my family was dying – and that someone was going to murder me.

The incessant chatter would drive me to my absolute limits, and I would use anything to try to quieten my mind, which invariably meant chemicals. I felt that they were the only way of putting an end to the turmoil within and relieving me of the feelings of acute stress and tension dominating my thoughts. I would use drugs to calm me down and then medicine to help me stay up, and that was the way it was throughout my early twenties. I was living in a state of perpetual fear – frightened even in my own home – and a cycle of ill health, which was an appalling way to be. Sometimes I would lie in my bed with my face constricted tight, wishing that someone would put an end to the torturous world I inhabited alone.

During the early 1990s fate intervened, and I was offered a new job and a career in Spain. I had become disillusioned by nursing, and although I was working only sporadically, I wondered if my job was to blame for my worsening condition. I seemed to be continuously looking for a reason to explain my depression. No matter what I did or how I did it, I desperately wanted to pull myself together and gain some clarity and control over my life. I had answered a advert in a newspaper for a travel consultant and felt sure that it would answer all of my problems. There was also scope for working abroad, which hastened my application, and I couldn't wait to have a new start.

Within a few weeks I had secured a position in Menorca and was confident that this would be my geographical cure and an end to my situation, which was deteriorating daily. Apart from the illness that was dominating my life, I was in a relationship with someone who had begun to use heroin. Given that I had an addictive nature, I was naturally concerned that I would be next in succumbing to the drug, and I couldn't wait to get away from it all and the people around me. My drinking was getting worse, and I would have memory blanks in which I was violent with anyone who happened to be around me. This, of course, was mortifying and would leave me feeling incredibly ashamed and embarrassed, as I genuinely couldn't remember what had happened. I was filled with self-hatred over my actions, and this fuelled my sense of inadequacy and, of course, increased my low mood. Sometimes I would be on the phone to the Samaritans long into the night, just desperate for help, and sometimes I would wonder where else there was left for me to turn as my situation grew more and more hopeless.

After the aircraft had landed, the sun shone down as I loaded my bags into the car; I really felt as though I had a chance to make the change in my life. I was so utterly convinced it would mean the end to my misery that I now wonder how I could have been so naïve. As the taxi drove through the pretty Menorcan villages, I remember feeling blessed that this opportunity had come my way, and I initially felt more in control of my feelings. However, within a few days of being there the mind-numbing flatness had returned, and as I waded through the surf I knew that it was all pointless. The water was the most beautiful turquoise and the fish would swim around my feet, but still I couldn't see what was before me as the evil mental chatter returned. My head would be filled with torment, and I couldn't see the paradise that surrounded me no matter how hard I tried. The people were lovely, the situation idyllic, and yet still the misery had followed me. I despaired as I realized that it was never going to leave me, no matter where I went or who I was with. As I looked out over the glorious cove, I remember feeling once again that I should give up and leave this world which I just didn't fit into.

By now I had seen several psychiatrists, numerous doctors, psychologists, counsellors and a good few gynaecologists, and not one of them had thought to ask me if my mood swings were related to my menstrual cycle. I had seen spiritualists and healers, and taken all sorts of medications in the hope that I would get better. I was a drug user and a borderline alcoholic, and I was suffering from all manner of emotional disturbances, which ranged from severe to catastrophic. I had tried art therapy, relaxation therapy and hypnosis to find a cure. I had moved house several times and even moved country in the hope that I would find some respite from the emotional misery that was, and is, clinical depression. By the time I left Menorca, I had been mentally ill for some seven years, and I was just twenty-two years old.

BILLY – 1990S
A FIRST-BORN SON AND A BONDING DELAY

During the early 1990s I was spending the long summer months in the Balearic Islands and reluctantly coming home for the winter. I experienced two hedonistic years in Ibiza where I met made some wonderful friends and could feel myself moving further away from my life in England. The Ibiza summers gave me some respite from the cold and monotony of living in the UK. As soon as I came home, the all too familiar gloom would descend on me and life would once again become unbearable. I felt as though Ibiza was my spiritual home, but there was only seasonal work there, which would force my return to England in the winter and increase my sense of melancholy.

Fortunately, during the winter of 1996 my colleagues and I were all offered new contracts which led us to the Canary Islands. This gave us all year-round employment and enabled me to finally give up my life in England for good. I stayed in Fuerteventura for some weeks, but unfortunately I didn't see eye to eye with the line manager, so quite quickly I decided to move to the next island, which was Lanzarote. It was the most beautiful evening as I boarded the ferry, with the volcanoes rising up majestically as the sun set over the sand dunes; I remember it as though it was yesterday. I had a sense of nervous excitement as I was going to an island where I didn't know a soul, and I'd had only had a brief conversation with the man who was to be my new team leader.

I was collected the following morning from my hotel. He drove up to the entrance in the most beautiful sports car and, as he introduced himself, I had a really good feeling about the place and immediately knew that I would stay there long term. It was completely different to anywhere I had ever been, and even though it didn't have the same perfect ambience as Ibiza, I liked it and felt as though I had finally found somewhere to settle. Unfortunately, my accommodation wasn't ready in time so I had to stay at the manager's house, which made me nervous to say the least. However, when we drove up to his villa my worries simply left me, and I was in awe of the place; it was quite simply stunning.

I could see that there was a vast amount of wealth surrounding me – I'd never seen anything like this place before. It was totally open plan in design, and in the middle was a huge sunken lounge with sumptuous cushions. As he showed me to my room he asked me if I wanted to use the sauna, and when he showed me the Jacuzzi and pool I started to feel amused at the situation I now found myself in. In the corner of the room I noticed two people, and he introduced me firstly to his girlfriend and then to James, who was to be my new line manager. I remember being surprised, as he looked a bit scruffy and not like manager material at all. However, as he shook my hand I stopped dead in my tracks: he had the most beautiful blue eyes I had ever seen and I blushed quite obviously, which made him smile. We sat down to dinner and I tried desperately not to make eye contact with him while trying to contain the butterflies in my stomach.

The months to come were wild and spontaneous, and within a few short weeks we fell madly in love. Although it wasn't intentional, I had felt an immediate connection and the fact that he was my manager made it all the more rebellious and exciting. All of my problems seemed to leave me as we spent every available minute together; he seemed to know exactly how to treat me. He took me for the most fabulous meals, we drank countless bottles of champagne and there seemed to be an abundance of money, which was often spent in the casino or on these opulent nights out. I was on a high for the next few months, having never before experienced such intensity and passion as I had for him. When we weren't out partying we were in bed making love, and I had an almost complete absence of depression, which was the first time in the whole of my adult life. I was just completely taken with him, and I hung on his every word. I even agreed to marry him and within a few short months we were making all manner of plans, which delighted my family and all those who knew us. It seemed as though I had found my soul mate, and he swore that he would look after me forever, which of course I believed.

As the heady months went on and I fell more and more in love, my broodiness increased, and in the summer of 1997 I became pregnant with my first child. James seemed delighted and if he had any doubts he never showed them; he even suggested that we should get married before the baby was born. I wanted to wait, as I didn't want to walk down the aisle with a bump and, anyhow, by the time I was six weeks pregnant I was suffering from dreadful morning sickness and unable to do anything. I was quite literally bedridden and the heat of the sun made me feel worse, so I was completely incapacitated. As the weeks went by I started to feel needy and tearful, and I so desperately wanted to feel well. As much as the doctor tried to convince me that it would pass, by the six-month mark I was still feeling dreadful, and I wondered if the nausea and exhaustion would ever leave me.

As I tried to nurture my growing baby and became more homely, James grew further away from me, and by the seventh month of my pregnancy the dynamics of our relationship had changed. The party-loving wild child in me had simply disappeared, and I had given up smoking and drinking as I desperately wanted to protect our baby. I so wanted to be a responsible parent but James couldn't break free from the lifestyle that we had both enjoyed. If we did go out, I had to come home halfway through the evening, which made him resentful, and I sensed a great change in his demeanour. I started feeling that we had made a mistake, and as the pregnancy progressed I could sense a great crack appearing in what had started as a whirlwind romance. This, of course, left me devastated, and I felt that my first and longed-for pregnancy was ruined.

He would say that he would be home at a certain time but fail or refuse to stick to his word. Eventually he stopped coming home at all and I wouldn't be able to get hold of him. This, of course, left me desperately worried, and I would pace the floor, trying to will his return. When he did appear I would be dreadfully tearful and this only pushed him further away. He started to disappear sometimes for days, and I became more and more desperate, wondering how I could have got him so wrong. Even though he was treating me badly, I was still trying to preserve the relationship, and to my shame I even begged him to stay with me and change his ways. I felt as though I was losing him and that he was deliberately pushing me away somehow. He would often create a situation to antagonize me, which would cause an argument of some kind, no matter how ridiculous. This would then give him licence to leave the house, regaining his sense of freedom and lack of responsibility, while I would be home alone and devastated.

As the birth of our baby approached, I could feel that all was lost and the stress was taking its toll on my system. I had a couple of scares at night, when I thought that the baby was coming and I couldn't reach James, which left me terrified and desperately isolated. I felt that I had no choice but to return to England to have the baby, as he clearly wasn't going to be there for me and I would have to go it alone. When I told him of my decision, I saw a look of relief come over his face, as this obviously freed him of any ties and allowed him to carry on with his own life regardless. Reluctantly, I packed as much as I could and he promised me he would follow in the weeks to come. As I boarded the aircraft and made my way home to my parents' house, I felt so disappointed that I was now pregnant 'on my own'.

Billy came into the world screaming and flailing his legs, with my mum by my side. Unfortunately, James didn't make the birth, which had been torturous and long, almost seventeen hours. As the midwife gave me my son, I was filled with regret that his daddy wasn't there. When he did arrive in the middle of the night, he seemed genuinely thrilled as he gazed at our baby who had inherited those piercing blue eyes. Billy seemed to recognize his daddy's voice, which I found fascinating, and as we were both taking him in, I could see the joy in James's face. I started to believe that maybe we had a chance – his bond with our son would help us secure a future. When we took Billy home to Mum's house, James seemed to be a proud daddy and was more than confident when helping me. I hoped it would last, as I was just so desperate to give our little boy the family life that he deserved.

Apart from the difficulties that James and I had experienced when I was pregnant, I had managed to stay 'depression-free'. This surprised me, and I felt sure that my illness had righted itself and those days were behind me. However, the birth of the baby hit me like a truck, and five days later I started to wonder what on earth I had done. Billy had terrible colic and seemed to be forever perched on my shoulder while I tried desperately to soothe him. He wouldn't feed properly and seemed to squirm when I held him against me. Nothing I did made it better and I was utterly exhausted and filled with anxiety as I tried everything I could think of to remedy the situation. I knew I had to get him settled before my return to Lanzarote, which I was dreading as I felt so poorly while trying to recover from the birth. I also felt cheated that the sudden rush of overwhelming love I had expected to feel had evaded me, and I couldn't tell anyone what I was really feeling. I went through the motions of caring for Billy but sometimes felt detached, as though he wasn't mine. I loved him but I didn't 'feel' him, which bothered me so much that I was certain that there must be something wrong with me.

I hoped that my feelings would change once I had Billy settled back in Lanzarote, but he continued to be in terrible pain back on the island. I tried so hard to console the poor little thing, but he would only stop crying when he was lying on my chest, so I was sleep deprived and unable to cope. James had already returned to his old ways and was barely at home, so there I was, lonely and desperate with a baby who simply didn't stop crying. The more he cried, the more I felt lost and overwhelmed, and my confidence was shaken. As the weeks went by a new set of symptoms arrived, and slowly but surely I relapsed back into depression.

At first it was so subtle and different from before that I almost didn't recognize it, and it sneaked up from a different angle, taking me by surprise. I began to feel impatient, and my irritability increased gradually and steadily as the weeks went by. If someone was speaking I would find it difficult to concentrate, and I would drift off mid-conversation as my mind struggled to maintain focus. When people were talking about any given subject, I would feel a wave of anger come over me, and I would hurry them to finish what they were saying. The people around me started to notice this, and my friend Claire said that I had lost my smile. This troubled me, as I had always managed to put on a brave front and had hidden my previous episodes from all who knew me. I desperately wanted people to think that I was a competent mother, and I felt ashamed and troubled that motherhood wasn't what I thought it would be. This new, mostly anger-orientated, set of symptoms I was experiencing would see me explode into rages which were completely unfounded and highly embarrassing. Whereas before, my illness had been sorrow-based, it had now changed and James remarked that I had turned into a 'right witch', making me feel even more self-conscious and incapable as a mother.

During the late summer of 1998 my life was in tatters. James and I finally split up for good – a combination of his dreadful behaviour and my increasing illness had left me unable to fight with him any more. As I boarded the plane home to England, I was broken-hearted, and I felt immeasurable guilt that I had robbed my baby of a normal family life, with a father. I had tried so hard to make it work, but I had nothing more to give. I knew returning to England wouldn't be easy, but I needed my family's help and support, which was something James wasn't prepared to give. As the plane took off for London and climbed over the clouds, my baby looked directly into my eyes and a sense of bereavement fell over me. Billy was by now just three months old, and he was simply quite beautiful.

Initially, I had to stay with my family, which was difficult to say the least as I felt as though I was imposing on them. Once I had secured accommodation for us, I did start to feel a little better, and I threw myself into looking after my baby, who was growing bigger by the day. His crying had got a little better, but I was still suffering from internalized anger, which I put down to the break-up and heartbreak I was feeling. I tried so desperately hard to bond with Billy, walking him in his pram while singing to him. I was hoping to feel the huge explosion of love that I imagined I was supposed to be feeling and that so many others had described. In fact, it was almost near his first birthday that I first noticed a sense of euphoria when I looked at him, and I finally started to feel like a real mummy with that unexplainable bond.

We had been settled in England for some time when I had another serious episode of loss of control. I had begun dating again and was desperate not to become pregnant, so I had visited the doctors in the hope of securing a permanent form of contraception. My thinking was that if I fell in love again it would relieve me of the sadness I felt over James. I still hadn't been able to get over our break-up and, despite it being some two years later, I would often dissolve into tears when thinking of him. As soon as I thought about him, I would be consumed with anger and a need for revenge that was intense and frightening. I would lie awake, wondering how on earth I could get over it, filled as I was with bitterness and hatred for him. I felt that Billy and I had been callously discarded into a life without a husband and a father, and I was grieving endlessly for my life in Spain and all of my friends. I couldn't seem to break free from the cycle of regret and pain. I felt sick to my stomach day in, day out, and sometimes I wondered if I would ever get over it or ever trust anyone again.

My appointment with the doctor resulted in me having the contraceptive injection, which I swear had a catastrophic effect on my mental state. Within a few hours of receiving it, my mental chatter had increased tenfold and I developed a huge knot in my stomach and felt dreadfully insecure. I started wailing and crying while lying on my bed, and I desperately tried to take hold of my feelings. Once again I had the ghostly feeling around me, and I grew terrified and would hyperventilate as I sobbed, while my baby looked on. I just didn't feel like me any more, and it was as if my thoughts had been planted there. It was like a monster had taken me over, and I was consumed with contempt for any living thing, including my son and anyone else who sprang to mind. Something dreadful had happened to me, and as I returned to the doctor later that week, I knew that I needed help and that my illness had returned. The intensity of my feelings was terrifying and sinister, and I couldn't calm down.

The next few months were filled with appointments as my mental state grew more serious and I became physically unwell. I really felt as though I were suffering from some mystery illness, as I seemed to be plagued by ill health and spent hours on the sofa. I had numerous infections, suffered extreme lower back pain, and developed acne on my back and pains in my joints. As much as I tried to explain it, the doctors were convinced that all of my problems were in my mind, a manifestation of the depression and anxiety. This increased my paranoia and I became convinced that they thought I was neurotic, even hypochondriac – and that I was imagining it all. Despite all of this, I asked the doctor for more help as I had realized that my symptoms were only there two weeks in a month, and were always followed by a menstrual period. Whatever my symptoms, whether they were irritability or panic attacks, they were a kind of prelude to my periods, which were once again causing me to feel faint and to sometimes vomit.

The doctor prescribed natural progesterone, which was known to help with premenstrual syndrome, and I prayed it would work. I was sick of feeling poorly and I was concerned that my illness would rub off on my baby, as I was so prone to losing my temper. Within a few minutes of using the progesterone, calm came over me and I immediately felt better. I couldn't believe it had happened so quickly, and at first I wondered if I was imagining it, as it was so instantaneous. I experienced the same feeling of serenity when I had a chilled glass of wine, and I could feel the medicine work its way through my system and through my veins. I used the progesterone regularly, and it was like finding a small miracle as the mood swings left me and my concentration returned. The terrible anger abated, and I felt an abundance of love as I cradled my little boy. As the days and weeks went by, I found a new spring in my step and the exhaustion left me, along with my rage and hostility.

By the time I realized that my illness was something to do with my hormones, I'd had numerous blood tests and ultrasound scans, and endless appointments with different health care professionals. I was suffering from severe depression and anxiety, and had developed multiple phobias, including of heights and flying. I was perpetually concerned about my health and worried that something would happen to my baby, whether it was murder or serious illness. Despite the initial reprieve that progesterone had provided, and the antidepressant medication I was using, I was still extremely poorly. Billy was four years old and I was thirty, and I had been ill for almost sixteen years, which was more than half my life.

That's when I started to visit the library, in the hope that I could find out where the doctors had failed and what on earth was wrong with me.

FREDDIE – 2003
A BRUSH WITH MADNESS AND A NEWBORN CHILD

I lost contact with James for four long years, and I tried desperately hard to get over him, although I still found myself pining at regular intervals. I would lie awake for hours, going over every minute detail to try to make some sense of the guilt and heartbreak that I felt, which seemed to be never-ending. Billy was approaching school age and my health was still compromised, with my menstrual difficulties continuing, so I was reading everything I could find on hormonal disturbances. I was diagnosed with polycystic ovary syndrome – my hunch was proved to be true – and that gave me some hope for the future. The consultant that I was seeing at the time decided to try a stronger contraceptive pill in the hope that it would regulate and ease my symptoms. However, I went on to have another relapse, which left me with severe panic attacks and yet more trips to the hospital's emergency department. My anxiety was so severe that I would often have to ask a friend to sit with me, as I felt so unsafe and insecure. I would hyperventilate and tremble violently, utterly convinced that I was going to die, and the experience would leave me feeling poorly for days after, with flu-like aches and pains.

After one particularly bad day, when I had one attack in the morning and another in the evening, I could see that my levels of anxiety had increased massively since I had started taking the pill. In fact, as much as the pill had eased some elements of my physical issues, it had had a catastrophic effect on my mental state, and I was certain it was responsible for this new panic disorder. I stopped taking it immediately and couldn't quite believe it when the anxiety stopped. Once again, I found myself trying to convince my own doctor that there was an issue with my hormones, but as much as I tried to explain everything to her, she still seemed sceptical, which was hugely frustrating and extremely demoralizing.

When Billy started school, his father and I resumed contact and I returned to Lanzarote for a holiday. Again, I was completely taken in by his charms and he wooed me with false promises and affection. He had a complete and profound hold over me, and Billy of course was delighted that he was at last able to meet his daddy. James managed to convince me that we had a future and that he wanted reconciliation, but it proved to be short-lived. Once I returned home he refused to take my calls, and I had no closure or any explanation. I just felt so sad for little Billy, who had told everybody about his new daddy only to be robbed of him yet again.

I had been home just two weeks, with no word from James, when I felt the all too familiar feeling low down in my pelvis. I knew I was pregnant, and my heart sank as the reality of the situation came over me. I simply couldn't believe that I had been so irresponsible as to let this happen, and I buried my head in my hands as I tried to contemplate the consequences. My friends said I was crazy for getting pregnant again, and one even offered to pay for a termination as she was so concerned about my state of mind. I didn't sleep for a week with the worry of it all, but as much as I knew my situation was hopeless, I realized that I wouldn't be able to cope with the guilt that an abortion would leave, and the long-term effect it would have on my already fragile disposition. In July 2003, I gave birth to my beautiful little Freddie, who was as calm and serene as a baby could be, and a delight to all who came to meet him.

Surprisingly, I had been extremely well throughout my pregnancy, without any depressive symptoms. This was something I had noticed with both pregnancies, and it intrigued me. Even though my situation seemed dire, I felt well and settled and even quite happy at times. Within a few hours of Freddie's arrival, I felt absolutely elated and excitable. I was totally in love with my baby and felt the overwhelming sense of love and protection that had been absent before. I wanted to shout out from the rooftops that my new baby had arrived, so over the moon was I with this new addition to my little family. Within a few short days I found that, as I went about my daily chores, I was over-efficient, methodical and hyperactive. Everything had to be done in a certain way and if my list of tasks wasn't completed by 9:30 at the latest, I would feel uncomfortable and agitated. I started to sing rather loudly and feel utterly joyous as I went about my day, which became more noticeable by those around me. Looking back, I was absolutely manic, and I seemed to be driven by a different energy that would sometimes leave me unable to sleep. I rushed from room to room, trying hard to burn it off even though it seemed to come from inside my head and not my body. Little did I know that this was a worrying sign of what was around the corner.

Freddie was just six weeks old when something terrible and unbelievable happened to me. Everything had been going well, too well, when I woke to feed the baby at six in the morning. As soon as I opened my eyes, I knew that something had gone dreadfully wrong, and for a moment I lay still, surveying my situation. When I tried to get out of bed, my body seemed to lock into position as if being held in a vice. My neck was so stiff

I wondered if I had suffered whiplash, and I struggled to make sense of how I was feeling. As I tried to move over to the crib, my legs seemed to give way and I stumbled across the room, unable to balance. As I moved my head to look around the room, it took my brain several moments to catch up, and I desperately tried to focus as a wave of terror took over me, my heart beating loudly in my chest.

I started to reason it out in my mind and decided that I must have mastitis, which can leave you feeling extremely unwell. As I made my way to the bathroom I realized that I was soaked through with sweat. I sat on the toilet and tried to remove my nightshirt, but as I did, I noticed that underneath my arms were lumps the size of small golf balls. What were they doing there? They had appeared overnight, and as I felt them I grimaced and struggled to bring my arms down, which had locked into position. I was in the most terrible pain and I cried out loudly. I tried to get a grip on the situation and return to my baby, who was by now crying for his feed. Breast milk began to pour over me, and I tried to move while the tears fell down my face onto my lap. Little Billy woke up and came into the room bewildered and half asleep, so I motioned to him to pass me the baby. As I tried to place Freddie onto my breast, I cried pitifully, wondering how on earth I would get out of this situation. I couldn't move my limbs properly and everything had seized up.

When the doctor came to see me she prescribed an antibiotic, and although I wasn't convinced that I had an infection I was so sick that I could barely be bothered to argue with her. I badly needed to sleep, but the baby wouldn't rest and Billy was home for the school holidays, desperate for my attention. As the day went on, my body grew so sensitive that the slightest touch would leave me wincing, and the tiniest noise would go right through me. Every time the baby cried or Billy spoke to me, it seemed as if the sound was magnified, and I covered my ears, trying to protect myself from what was almost a physical pain. I felt so acutely on edge that any sound left me feeling as though someone was scraping their fingers down a blackboard or crunching on a piece of silver foil. When teatime came, I was trying so desperately hard to function that I became almost robotic and shifted around aimlessly, lost in another world. I felt so acutely strange, it seemed as though something else had over taken my personality, and I grew frightened at this new and disturbing symptom, which left me convinced that I would never be the same again.

Over the course of the next few days, my mind tipped into psychosis and I lost myself entirely. At first I wondered if I had a temperature and was perhaps delirious, but as the hours went by I knew it was something far more serious. As I lay on the bed, I pleaded with God to put me to sleep and help me stop feeling so poorly. I could see the baby in his crib while the half-light seemed to lull me into the deepest sleep. Suddenly, I felt a huge jerk and, as I jumped, I wondered what was happening. I was flooded with panic and heard a loud chugging noise in my ears, which became quite deafening. What could it be? Where was it coming from? As I tried to fathom where the sound was coming from, it dawned on me that there had to be a tractor in my bedroom, and as I turned to see where it was, I realized that I couldn't move. My whole body was completely and utterly paralysed, and when I say that, I mean it in every sense. Despite my best efforts, I couldn't move a single inch of my body, and I was now floating upwards towards the ceiling. The noise buzzed louder and I was pulled from the umbilicus straight up; I was powerless to stop it. I tried to make a sound and a groaning noise seemed to escape, but by then I was observing myself from above, looking down on my own bedroom. I could clearly see my own motionless body on the bed, and everything around me, but I didn't belong to myself and had left my own body. I tried to pull myself back down to the bed, but my body seemed to be held by an invisible magnet against the ceiling. I remember thinking, 'Don't panic, it's just a dream,' but as I thought it I knew that it wasn't true and that something supernatural was happening to me. I spent what seemed like an eternity suspended in the air while I attempted to cry out for help, but I couldn't say anything.

The fear that I felt was something I hadn't experienced before. I genuinely believed that I had reached another dimension, and I was now in a different and terrifying world. It was so alien and unearthly that I was quite sure I had lost my mind and would never recover or come back to myself. Just as I started to believe that I would stay in the air for ever, I seemed to snap back and be lying on the bed once again. With a loud gasp I became aware of my surroundings and that Billy was standing at my side. I pulled him in beside me and held him tight for comfort. As I lay awake, rigid with fear and too scared to go back to sleep, I tried to convince myself that I had suffered from a bizarre nightmare, even though, deep down, I was as scared as anyone could be, and I knew that something inside me had changed.

In the morning I felt quite traumatized, and despite my best efforts to put the experience to the back of my mind, I felt disturbed and frightened all day. I had to go through to the kitchen, as I didn't want Billy to see me crying and in such obvious distress. A friend offered to watch him so that I could take an afternoon nap with the baby, but when I finally got off to sleep I had the most awful dream in which I murdered my children. I was chopping up their little bodies and desperately trying to hide the parts so that I wouldn't be found out. When I woke I was more disturbed than ever and kept breaking down and crying for my mum. I was clutching myself as everything hurt, but the hurt was coming from my mind, which seemed to be attached to a knot inside my stomach. I felt lost and alone and deeply insecure, with even the floor seeming uneven beneath my feet, which made me stumble around, unable to balance.

As evening approached, the feeling worsened and a sickening nausea was building inside me. I decided that if I did something 'normal' then I would feel 'normal', so I dressed the boys and drove to the supermarket in the hope that it would help me get a grip on my emotions. As we walked round the shop, I noticed that the lights seemed far too bright and, again, it seemed as though all my senses were heightened. I could really see how colourful everything was, and yet somehow the glare was too much for my eyes. The colours were so vivid and true that I felt sure they weren't normally like that, and I tried to close and shelter my eyes. I did my best to ignore what I was feeling and seeing, but I grew confused and lost my bearings as I walked down the aisles. As my disorientation continued I slipped into a trance-like state, and things that were normally familiar to me I simply didn't recognize. What was I doing here and where was I? What was happening to me?

As I tried hard to compose myself I seemed to go into a dream state, in which I wasn't sure if I was awake or not. My body felt numb and everything seemed artificial, as if I was in my very own cartoon or a colourful book. All around me seemed plastic, and there were beings that I didn't recognize floating past me. I was totally perplexed by this, and once again I seemed to be in another dimension as I surveyed what was going on around me. I looked down at the children in the trolley, and as my mouth grew dry and my heart pounded in my chest, I knew that I was very ill and needed help. I looked at my arms and held them up to the light. As I squinted from the brightness of everything, I felt that my hands were somebody else's and didn't belong to me. As I tried to use them I didn't recognize them as mine, and I grew detached and separated from myself, as though I were watching a film. Once again, I moved from out of myself and observed the whole scene from far away, looking down on us all from outside my own body.

When I finally 'came around', I realized that the beings floating by were actually other shoppers and, of course, the staff. One lady looked at me with real pity in her eyes, which was enough to make me feel that she would grab my children, so I removed them from the trolley and fled. As I buckled them into the car I was convinced we were in imminent danger; I was running for my life and the lives of my children. As we drove home the boys began to cry, and I immediately started to trance out again. The street lights seemed so bright I could barely see, and I suddenly seemed to be in a dodgem car at a fair … everything had changed! The road ahead was computerized, and as I rushed to finish the race, I knew that I was losing it. I thought I was in a simulator, and I couldn't for the life of me work out what was real and what was imagined, or where the dream ended and reality began.

As we got home I clutched the boys firmly to me and tried to figure out what was wrong. I was incredibly frightened as the magnitude of what was happening to me began to take hold. I ran around the whole flat closing the curtains, but I was so paranoid that I felt sure someone might have got in with us, so I kept every light on. Trying to get the children bathed and into bed was a huge challenge, but finally, as I laid the baby in his crib, I was able to reflect on what had happened. As I looked at his eyes, a creeping nausea came over me – he looked so strange and different. I tried to focus on him but his eyes became spirals that bore into me, twisting and turning. I moved away from him, unable to look, but I knew I would have to hold him, so I carefully picked him up. As I pulled him close, I retched violently and vomit filled my mouth, which I then swallowed. As he squirmed against me I gave a shudder. It felt as though I was holding a giant insect, which was now writhing its body against me, and it took everything in my power not to throw him against the wall. I actually visualized that moment in my mind, and imagined his skull breaking in two.

As I shouted out for someone to help me, I tried to carry on holding him, but I just couldn't do it. He smelled absolutely rancid and not like my baby at all, so I had to put him down. As I turned my face away from him, he knew what I was thinking and he was as suspicious of me as I was of him. Just the thought of holding him filled me with disgust, and I curled my knees up to my chest and rocked. It felt so soothing just to sit there and sway, and when the tears came I sobbed long into the night, with the baby beside me, who didn't look like a human baby at all. As I sat cross-legged on my bed, scared to open my eyes, the ache in my legs was so violent I wondered if I might die. The stabbing pains in my breasts were so brutal I felt sure that they might kill me, and my mental anguish was so great that I just wished I would hurry up and die, as I had finally and definitely gone mad.

Trying to care for the children the next day was an absolute nightmare. I simply tried to be normal and held the parasite baby as little as possible because it made the feelings I was experiencing much worse. When I tried to bath him I would avert my gaze, as it felt too odd to look at him. By the evening, however, the feeling would return with a vengeance. It was always the same pattern of events, with the creeping nausea and internal shuddering that would quite often leave me holding on to the walls for balance. Everything would start to look and feel strange, and the flat itself wouldn't look familiar, but instead creepy and eerie, as If I had walked into my very own horror movie. Everything was so visually distorted and twisted, it didn't look like my home at all, and I wondered who had changed everything. Who did it all belong to, or was it really mine?

Once I had got the children to bed, I would lie on my bed, panting with fear while waiting for the inevitable feeling to take over. Sometimes I would drift off to sleep, but my nightmares were so bad that I would always wake up crying, convinced that we were all dead. By the fourth night I woke to find my friend

Katie standing at the end of the bed, which was extraordinary as it was gone midnight and I'd been in bed some time. I was just so confused by her being there, and as I asked her what she was doing in my room, she pulled out the biggest dragonfly I had ever seen from behind her back. It was all the colours of the rainbow and was opening and shutting its wings as if ready to fly. She pulled another from her other side and it was equally beautiful but smaller than the first. As she held them up proudly, she seemed to be smiling at me in a sarcastic kind of way, and as she mocked me, she fed one dragonfly to the other, as if performing some kind of magic trick. Of course, I was mortified by this horror unfolding in front of me, and as I hid under my quilt, I begged her to leave me alone.

I couldn't work out whether I was asleep and dreaming or whether it was all actually happening. Sometimes I felt completely unable to move but was aware of my surroundings; I felt a pressure keeping me on the bed and a strange roaring in my ears. This, of course, left me a bit stuck, so I lay central on the bed to prevent anything getting to me.

Despite my situation, I cottoned on to the fact that I was hallucinating, even though it all seemed so real. I tried closing my eyes, hoping that the visions would go away, but when my eyes were closed I would have pop-up visions instead. Sometimes they were in black and white and sometimes they were quite colourful, fluorescent even, which would again hurt my eyes. Sometimes they were friendly and quite pretty, and other times they were menacing, which of course would scare me out of my wits.

Despite my irrationality, at times I was quite with it and knew I was mentally ill. I even wondered if I had become schizophrenic or had been taken over by somebody else, an imposter within me. As my thoughts progressed, I started to feel that it would be better to have the boys adopted, as I was too ill to look after them and I wanted to save them from more pain. It seemed the best thing for all of us and, as I started to plan it all in my head, I decided quite rationally that I would make the necessary arrangements once I had seen my doctor. I would find a family to take care of them and they would go to a new and loving home without a poorly mummy who couldn't look after them.

The drive to the mental health clinic the next day was hard because I lost my way there, even though it was within walking distance of my house. By now I was disassociating so regularly that I was barely able to function. The psychiatric nurse could immediately see the severity of my condition and said I needed to see the duty psychiatrist, which came as a huge relief. As I was talking to her, I started to hallucinate in her office. She made me hold my baby, which made me squirm and cry, and as I returned him to his pram, I turned him away from me, unable to look into his eyes. I was utterly convinced that she was out to harm me. I felt so frightened when I held him and I felt sure that my body was physically repelling him. As I explained what I was feeling, she immediately diagnosed post-natal depression, which I simply didn't believe, and I argued with her relentlessly. I was trying to convey the fact that I wasn't depressed and sometimes even felt elated, but this seem to convince her even further that I really was unwell.

On that particular day sitting in that office with the doctor and my baby conspiring against me, was without doubt the lowest point of my life. I wanted to crawl under her desk and fade away. It was as though every cell in my body had broken into a thousand little pieces, with nothing more to give. To look at my darling Freddie, whom I loved with every ounce of my being, and not be able to think of him as mine. To be convinced that I had given birth to a stranger whom I didn't recognize.

The psychiatrist sent me on my way with a packet of antidepressants and a sedative to help me sleep. Reluctant as I was to stop breastfeeding, once little Freddie latched on I would immediately disassociate, so he needed to have formula feeds. He took to them straightaway and throughout all of my disturbances he was quite simply the model baby. This obviously compounded my feelings of guilt and shame, which have never left me. Initially, I couldn't tell anyone what I had been experiencing, but I was being heavily sedated so a friend came to help me with the night feeds. I had intermittent moments of lucidity but also times when I would panic and be frightened for no apparent reason. The feelings and sensations I felt were so bizarre I began to think I would be stuck with them forever.

The night the antidepressant began to work I remember well, as I was able to hold the baby without feeling odd and dreamlike. It had taken roughly three weeks, but I started to feel different and slowly more at ease. I wanted to hold the baby and he seemed like mine again. I started to look forward to feeding time and I didn't squirm as I held him, or feel frightened and suspicious.

This initial respite, however, was all too short, and some six weeks after I had stopped breastfeeding I suffered a serious relapse, with a return of the nightmares and horrendous visions when I closed my eyes. It was so sudden I was completely taken aback and I couldn't believe it was happening again. My moods swung violently, and I felt absolutely murderous towards everyone and everything. Within a few days I knew once again that something had gone wrong, and in desperation I called the postnatal depression helpline. I had been so utterly convinced that I was better, and when the lady on the phone explained that I was probably going to have a period, and this was the reason for this sudden relapse, it was a huge light-bulb moment. Within a day or so I had indeed started, and the episodes of strangeness passed as suddenly as they had arrived.

The lady on the helpline sent me an information pack, and when it arrived I started to read every available piece of information and all the suggested books. I was furious when I learned that I was supposed to have continued using my progesterone therapy after the birth of my baby, and I couldn't believe that my own doctor hadn't reminded me. It is a known fact that women who suffer from hormonal disturbances can use progesterone as a preventative in the post-natal period, when hormone levels can radically plummet. The more I used my suppositories, the calmer I became, and the more I read, the more I learned about the effect our hormones can have on our mental health. I was livid that such a valuable piece of information had been overlooked, and I could barely contain my resentment towards my medical team.

No sooner had I realized the connection than it became more and more obvious, and I would have a monthly mini-psychosis, which was extremely frightening and all-consuming. As soon as I started to ovulate, the mad woman would move in and take over my life. Week by week I was plagued by delusions, paranoia, nightmares, daymares and an exhausting list of symptoms so severe that they had a disastrous effect on my personality. The fact that it was so avoidable was even harder to bear, but the reality was that my body had been so sensitive to the sudden drop in hormones after giving birth that it had created a type of chemical chaos which now seemed to be incurable. The situation was affecting my body chemistry to such an extent that not only was I mentally fragile, my physical health was also appalling with endless infections and compromised immunity. Sometimes I had a kind of vertigo with terrible shaking attacks and episodes of stumbling.

By the time little Freddie was two, I was still sick. In fact by then I had been poorly for over half of my life and I wondered if I would ever be taken seriously again.

CODY – 2010 THE LONG-TERM STRUGGLE WITH HORMONAL ILLNESS

In the spring of 2005, I took the boys for a holiday to Tenerife for a much-needed break, after what had been a terrible two years. I had turned a considerable corner and was using antidepressants and progesterone therapy, along with a three-hourly starch diet to stop my episodes of low blood sugar which seemed to make any underlying symptoms considerably worse. Sometimes I would wake up in the night with a racing mind and unwanted thoughts, so I would get up and have a snack. If I didn't, I would have palpitations and anxiety attacks, so as much as I knew I wasn't cured, I did understand the illness and all of its manifestations.

I also cottoned on to the fact that tiredness and stress were quite simply my worst enemies, so I would still sleep in the daytime. If I didn't take a nap, by the early evening I simply wouldn't be able to cope – I'd feel desperate and overwhelmed. I was also still suffering from brain fog and dementia-like episodes, when the slightest task (counting money, for example) would leave me completely perplexed and confused. This, of course, heightened my irritability, and I would sometimes scream out with the sheer frustration of my never-ending symptoms. Although I was greatly improved in comparison to when Freddie was born, I was still very poorly whenever my period approached. This left me dreading my own monthly cycle, and sometimes, even though I felt sure I had reached rock bottom, there was still lower to go. Once I had been through a period I would be OK again and the normal me would return almost as if the whole bizarre episode hadn't happened. I knew immediately when the cycle would start as I would become so sensitive to sound, and some noises would trigger me so badly and were almost painful.

On my return home from Tenerife on a crisp and beautiful spring morning, I bumped into an old friend who worked as a gardener in our neighbourhood. I hadn't paid much attention to Den previously, but as we chatted on this particular day I realized that he had the loveliest kind eyes and I was somehow drawn to him. I felt like I needed some adult company and asked him out, which was very out of character for me. Within a couple of days we went on a date, and he took me to a lovely restaurant where we chatted easily and endlessly. It was a strange situation because I didn't feel attracted to him in a romantic sense, but I did feel a bond with him – and he had the added bonus of making me laugh, which was just what I needed at the time. Even though I didn't fancy him (and he didn't me), I suddenly wondered at the table if he was the man I would marry. This seemed altogether quite strange and I dismissed it, not really wanting to get heavily involved, given that I was a single parent with excessive emotional and psychological baggage.

As the months went by he also showed himself to be the most wonderful friend to the boys, and in particular to Freddie, with whom he bonded immediately. Initially, I was very guarded about this and concerned that they would become too close, so I cooled things off a few times as I was worried that the boys would get hurt. Quite simply, I didn't trust anyone, good or bad, and my illness was still dominating my thoughts and clouding my judgement. I was just so worried about every tiny thing in every tiny way, and my anxiety and health worries were always there. At times I was so obsessed with getting better and being a good mummy that there didn't seem to be anything else left to give anyone, and I found it quite hard having somebody else around me. Despite this, we stayed together and Den went on to accompany me to every appointment, no matter what it was, so desperate were we to find a cure.

During the Christmas of 2008 we were married in a beautiful winter ceremony, and I just felt delighted and very blessed that I had found someone so supportive and kind. The wedding was conducted by candlelight, and I just felt so overwhelmed and in love with him. His patience and understanding had totally won me over, and he adopted the boys the very next year, which filled me with the deepest respect. Much as I was joyful and fulfilled by my new marital status, my depression was always lurking in the background and sometimes still managed to take me by surprise. Despite my knowledge and understanding of the hormonal elements of my condition, I would still have immense temper tantrums and overreact to the slightest situation. This would leave me hysterical and unable to calm down, sometimes for several hours. I knew I was doing it but was simply unable to stop, and I was so irrational I would sometimes even pick an argument without knowing why. These blow-ups were so intense they would frighten the children, and I would be left with a great deal of shame and guilt in the days that followed.

As the months went on, I tried desperately hard to balance my hormones, but sometimes I would forget to take my medication and then have an almighty outburst, sometimes so serious that I would have to run away. This would, of course, leave Den frantic with worry and filled with hopelessness, which then fuelled my sense of remorse and hatred of my condition. I would therefore spend two weeks spreading misery while in the late luteal phase and then the following two weeks trying to make up for all the things I had said and done wrong. On one particular day I had smashed up the bathroom and attempted to drive off in my car when Den stepped in my way and I accidently clipped him with the wheels of the car. Afterwards I was absolutely horrified by my behaviour which worsened more and more each month. It all seemed so draining, and we both felt absolutely powerless to stop something that seemed to be dominating our whole lives.

During the first year of our marriage we also had the dilemma of whether to have another baby, and the risks associated with that. Of course we both wanted to have a child of our own, but the enormity and severity of my condition simply couldn't be ignored, and sometimes I wondered if I could ever face the personal agony of another psychosis, and indeed the suicide risks. There were times when I had every intention of ending it all and I felt completely out of control of my own emotions. My fight or flight response was so highly activated; the slightest issue would leave me over-catastrophizing and off I would run for the hills.

As my knowledge of my condition increased, and our longing for a child intensified, we started to look at alternative therapies in the hope that we could strengthen my weakened immunity. I started to get attacks of shingles and I also began to suffer from migraines with a full and complete visual aura. It was so frightening to see what I was becoming and I just felt so guilty. Den was doing more and more and I was doing less and less, so increasingly he was becoming the main breadwinner and a house husband.

We decided to seek out holistic remedies, and we spent a fortune on alternative healing as well as an organic diet. At one point I was seeing a cranial osteopath, a homeopath and a Reiki healer. I tried reflexology and started to use Bach Flower Remedies in the hope that they would at least lessen my symptoms. The chronic fatigue and joint flare-ups would be so debilitating I would have to sleep and at one point I was spending the majority of the day in bed or on the sofa.

Everything helped to begin with, including the meditation and deep prayer that I was trying, but after a while they would lose their efficacy and I would be back to square one. It was costly and time-consuming, but mostly I was just so sick of it all. I was sick of being sick, I was sick of researching and sick of being me, really. After everything that I'd tried, I was starting to give up hope of ever achieving full remission, which of course increased my despair, and at times even exacerbated my condition.

Despite all this, the psychiatrist was happy for me to try for another baby, and didn't seem the slightest bit concerned that I was using high-dose medication to keep me stable. However, he wanted me to try Cognitive Behavioural Therapy (CBT) to see if it might lessen my symptoms. This I did, going on a ten-week course with a psychological therapist, and I relished what I found to be the most effective treatment I'd tried so far. I had to be taught a whole new way of thinking, but it gave me a new weapon against my illness, and in particular my mental chatter which was absolutely relentless.

With CBT I had to write down every little thought and challenge the unhelpful ones. The therapist was so kind and professional but the homework she gave me was so intense it often left me feeling triggered. Despite this, I persevered and eventually was able to understand that the abnormal and suicidal thoughts were the illness thinking for me, and not some part of my own personality. This powerful therapy was so effective at addressing my mental state that it also helped me make sense of my depersonalization and strange episodes that had been following me around since puberty. As unpleasant as they were, I was able to understand that they would indeed pass and were only a temporary sensation.

With the help and guidance of the mental health team, Den and I decided to bite the bullet and try for another baby. We had a wonderful delayed honeymoon cruising around the Mediterranean and in March 2010 our darling little Cody was born.

During my pregnancy, there had continued to be an absence of symptoms. This in itself was staggering to me, and I felt better than I had done in many years. However, despite the obstetricians saying that there were no problems in using antidepressant medication during pregnancy, Cody was suffering from the withdrawal of the medication that had crossed the placenta. When he was taken to special care, I noticed that his breathing was laboured and he was jerking and sneezing, which was an obvious concern. The paediatrician also refused to let me breast-feed him as there was a chance it could lead to pulmonary hypertension in Cody. Discovering this was such a shock to us, and Den and I felt that the doctors hadn't been forthcoming with this information. We were beside ourselves with worry while little Cody had to stay in hospital until the medication had cleared from his system. As we gazed at our little baby, I was once again filled with a sense of guilt that my illness had affected him so badly. I couldn't help but feel that I had let him down, and also that we had been let down by the team looking after us. I even questioned my desire and longing for another child, knowing that I probably wouldn't have gone ahead if I'd known this would happen. Even though they had warned me that there might be some mild issues when Cody was born, I certainly hadn't realized how serious they could be. Yet again our happy event was clouded in a sense of misery as we anxiously waited for him to come home.

In the weeks that followed Cody's birth, I used progesterone suppositories at every opportunity to prevent the sudden drop in hormones that I was so sensitive to. I stuck rigidly to the three-hourly starch diet and refused to allow myself to get overtired. I would sit down as much as I could and put myself and the baby above everything else. When I was woken in the night, I would use some progesterone and have a snack, and initially I saw no signs of my previous problems. Cody seemed to suffer no long-term ill effects, but he did struggle with colic for nine months, which was challenging to say the least. However, it felt so different having the love and support of a husband, and I tried to make the most of every moment, knowing that Cody would be my last child.

By the time Cody was six months old my periods had returned and my symptoms were back with a vengeance. At first I tried desperately to 'think' my way out of it but day by day, and month by month, different noises magnified and I also started to smell things that weren't there, which was a new and disturbing symptom. Quite suddenly I would smell urine or even strong perfume and even have the taste in my mouth afterwards, which was deeply unpleasant. These olfactory hallucinations often coincided with more pop-up visuals, which were also increasing with alarming speed. At one point I saw a horrible mutant mermaid with huge claws, which was absolutely terrifying. Another particularly disturbing vision was of people in gas masks coming towards me when I closed my eyes. Sometimes I would see spirals and sometimes animals would materialize in the sky or sometimes on the curtain rail in my bedroom. Even though I knew they weren't real, it was so dreadful knowing what my hormones were capable of doing to me.

Despite being on various forms of medication as the months went by, everything I threw at my illness seemed to be working less and less. If I had a bad back, for example, it would always be worse in the week before my period. If I caught a simple cold or sore throat, it would inevitably be at that time. My whole body seemed to have an allergic reaction to my cycle. I would be irritable, agitated and an absolute nightmare to live with. This, of course, was all the more unbearable because I desperately wanted to look after my family but was unable to do so. People around me also noticed my mood swings and would pass comment on the number of times I was taken ill and rushed into hospital. Sometimes I would be so despairing of my menstrual cycle that I would beg my doctor for help while she looked at me blankly, not knowing what else to suggest. The situation was simply intolerable, and by the time Cody was just a few months old I had once again begun to lose my fight, with suicide seeming the lesser of the two evils.

My pursuit of a cure took on a different meaning quite suddenly during the autumn of 2010. I read in a newspaper about Professor John Studd, a specialist in London who had done new and vital research on my condition. He had retired from medical practice but he had colleagues who he had trained personally and would be able to help me. Mr Nick Panay had an amazing reputation in treating all manner of hormonal problems and, despite the distance between his consulting rooms and my home, I was able to secure a referral. Why I hadn't been referred before was another mystery, but I was so pleased to have found a specialist NHS clinic that I counted the days until my appointment. By the time it came around I had researched Mr Pannay thoroughly and was in awe of this man who had helped so many women. Many of them were far worse than me and this gave me us immense hope for the future.

As Den and I waited anxiously in the waiting room to be called, I prayed so hard that this would be the break that we needed. My recent and sudden decline was leaving us absolutely desperate, but I knew that if anyone could help me conquer my reproductive depression it would be this particular doctor. We had exhausted every other avenue and wasted so much time and money seeking out different remedies that we were both reaching the end of our rope. Den wasn't coping, I had long given up coping and the day-to-day concept of living and being so poorly was simply unmanageable. I couldn't go on and the thought of being the way I was until menopause was simply horrifying. I would rather have been dead. Den knew this, I knew this and, when I told Mr Panay my story from beginning to end, he immediately understood. He was the first doctor I had seen who requested a blood test to look at my hormonal profile. He was also the first doctor in some thirty years who knew all about reproductive depression.

HYSTERECTOMY – 2012
THE QUEST FOR A CURE AND THE STARTLING RESULT

Having a depressive illness, whether it is hormonal or otherwise, is a very difficult thing to explain, especially if you have never had personal experience of it. This in itself often left me feeling alienated as I struggled to articulate my illness to others, who would often look at me with a blank expression. As sick as I was of the whole situation, I also realized that I was becoming a tremendous bore thanks to my obsession with my condition. My psychiatrist's insistence that I was bipolar was all the more frustrating, and he still couldn't explain why I was only 'bipolar' for two weeks of every month. Once I had found the correct doctors, however, I was so relieved to know that help was available and I could be treated.

Within a month or so the blood tests had revealed a great deal, more than I had anticipated. I had always thought that the genetic fault lay in my progesterone levels, but the test results were saying that my oestrogen levels were also undetectable in my bloodstream. This was a revelation to us all and gave new insight into how and why my body was simply unable to function properly. In short, I had a colossal problem which would never have got better without medical intervention. Using antidepressants and a mood stabilizer was helping but it was as if my body was a car that was driving without the petrol. Even though female hormone levels can fluctuate a great deal, my body was reaching a state of crisis every month and this was having a catastrophic effect on both my immunity and my mental health.

The blood test revealed I was also low in folate and iron which meant I was anaemic, the result being my dizziness and vertigo. The hormonal sensitivity which is now known as premenstrual dysphoric disorder (PMDD), or even late luteal phase dysphoric disorder, was only likely to become worse as I approached the menopause. This left me in a state of profound terror as I contemplated a life where I could possibly even get worse. I just couldn't think how I would survive it and, once more, whether my marriage would.

Mr Pannay gave me a prescription for an oestrogen patch, and I started to use it immediately. At first I was reluctant to try it, as I was worried that it might contain a synthetic hormone that had previously sent me over the edge. Once Mr Pannay had reassured me that the hormones were bioidentical, so they worked just the same as my own hormones, I was able to use the patches without a sense of anxiety, and I couldn't wait to feel the response. The reality was that without using them, I was unlikely to get better, and as he had treated thousands of women over the years I felt a sense of hope. I still needed to use the natural progesterone as it would protect my womb, but the patches allowed my body to receive the necessary hormones in a controlled and steady dose, rather than in the fluctuations that were causing my body to react in such a critical way.

Within a month or so, the patches had breathed some life back into me and I felt much improved. I was more in control of my own thoughts and I had a whole month without suffering from an attack of shingles. My joint flare-ups also settled down, and the lower back pain I had experienced since I was a teenager simply left me. However, I had been down this road before, and much as I wanted this new intervention to work, I didn't want to be lulled into a false sense of security. I remained guarded and was forever waiting for a relapse. Mr Pannay had warned me that, as I was often suicidal, I was a more serious case and would probably need a hysterectomy and my ovaries removing to turn off the whole system completely. He explained that in the long term this would create a 'blank canvas' that would see me rely on natural hormonal therapy rather than my own hormones, which I clearly couldn't metabolize correctly. It seemed that the illness had become so entrenched it could still only be 'managed', and I wasn't cured in the conventional sense. I would have to continue to take things day by day, or rather month by month. This was my life now and I had to accept that it was a long term strategy rather than an instantaneous cure.

I had been using oestrogen therapy for many months, along with progesterone, when I had a sudden relapse with huge repercussions. No matter how often these relapses occurred I was always totally surprised by them, and despite my incessant research they always came without any warning. Again I tried to 'think the thoughts away'. This particular episode was aggressive and as I looked in the mirror at my own reflection I couldn't quite believe what I was seeing.

As I gazed at the person looking back at me, I didn't recognize myself and I jumped at the sight of what was before me. I looked so different and odd, and I was sure I must be dreaming. I bit down on my lips, tried to compose myself but when I closed my eyes I saw a strange little lady who didn't appear to have any legs. I knew immediately it was happening again. Even though I had used the hormones properly, it seemed that no matter what I threw at it, the condition itself was more powerful than anything I could use to treat it.

As the weeks went by I increased my medication and tried every conceivable holistic therapy in the hope that it would lessen the symptoms. Once again, I had the compulsion to sleep and sometimes felt as weak as a rag doll. The simplest task would take a colossal effort and I felt as though I was walking through treacle. My nightmares were back with a vengeance as well as the suicidal thoughts. These compounded my feelings of guilt and self-hatred. Sometimes I felt so anxious and unsafe that I was convinced I had truly lost my mind. As I spent more and more time in bed I felt like the mad woman who lived at the top of the house with no hope for the future.

During the spring of 2012 my declining health was at its greatest and I had finally run out of options. Confiding in my husband that I was having suicidal thoughts again and wasn't to be trusted, we both knew that the time had come. We didn't tell a single soul for fear of anyone influencing my decision, and I made the appointment and asked for a referral for a hysterectomy. By now the fatigue and the fibromyalgia were so bad I was almost embarrassed to tell people for fear of them thinking I was a malingerer.

When I met the surgeon we looked through my menstrual charts and she agreed wholeheartedly that time was of the essence. I had tried every conceivable way to cure myself, but it just wasn't meant to be. Once we had discussed my options I began to feel empowered, and my research, combined with her knowledge, told me that it just might work. By now I was in touch with other sufferers so I knew that this last option could give me my life back.

Although I would have preferred to have the operation sooner rather than later, the surgeon wanted to switch off my hormonal system by injection first to see how I would feel. This would prepare me for surgery and give me a good idea of what to expect once I was plunged into 'surgical menopause'. This injection was to be given every three months and I was dreading it more than the hysterectomy itself. I was so concerned that I would suffer an abnormal reaction that I really didn't want to have it done. I was already so unstable, and I was terrified that it would cause a disturbance in me that I wouldn't recover from. I went over and over everything in my mind, trying to consider every possible outcome, which of course fuelled my existing anxiety. What if I fell into another psychosis? What if it didn't work at all and I had been wrong all along? What if I ended up being sectioned and leaving my children?

On the day I had the injection, my legs were trembling uncontrollably as I entered the doctor's surgery. The nurse was so kind to me, and she explained that the injection was an implant that would shrink my womb in preparation for surgery, allowing the whole procedure to be done by keyhole. As the needle went in, straight through my tummy, I remember feeling absolutely sick of it all. I was sick of the tests, sick of being ill, sick of talking about it and sick of thinking about it. I bit down hard on my lip to try to stay in control, but when I got up to leave the room afterwards the nurse passed me a tissue. Once I got into the car I cried bitter tears, as I was far more scared of what the injection might do to me than of having a major operation. The endless anguish and misery, the worry of it all and the abject fear that I might have made my whole situation worse was just something that I couldn't even contemplate. I drove slowly home and cried all the way.

Within a couple of hours of having the jab I felt a transition that I hadn't experienced before, and it felt very odd. At first I wondered if it was just a coincidence or if I was imagining it, but as I went about my day I knew for certain that something was happening. Before collecting the children I went to the supermarket, and as this was something that often filled me with dread I was already expecting a wobble. Although the injection had been painful at the time, once I had finished browsing the shelves of the supermarket, the soreness had passed and I had forgotten all about it. Instead, a warm calm had subtly come over me, and a new serenity enveloped my whole body. The knot that had permanently lived in my stomach for the last twenty-odd years had slowly started to unravel and the tension was leaving my body. At first I wondered what this feeling was, and even whether it could be psychosomatic, but when I got to the checkout I realized that I was being 'switched off'. The simplest task such as unloading the shopping would normally leave me exasperated and confused, but this time it was absolutely surreal, and a feeling of great comfort fell over me.

I efficiently unloaded the trolley without the usual mental chit-chat that had been part of me for so long, and as I counted the money I felt nothing unpleasant at all. I didn't feel panicked, I didn't feel lost and the usual brain fog simply wasn't there. I was smoother and more controlled, without a hint of the usual emotional turmoil. I was cool, calm and completely at ease with the situation I was in, and this mundane chore, which would normally cause me so much pain and emotional despair, was the easiest and most natural thing in the world. Normally I would feel so fretful and uneasy that I would have a sense of paranoia that I was being watched by an outside source but, this time, all of that was absent. For the first time ever I could go about my day without feeling aggressive and hostile, and the change was simply miraculous.

Feeling like a 'normal' person was absolutely wonderful, and it only hastened my desire to have the operation. The injection had such a radical effect that I couldn't wait to get rid of this major organ that had caused me so much pain and misery; my initial fear of being switched off for good had been totally unfounded. As the weeks went by the injection would wear off and then I couldn't wait to receive the next one, as the effect was so calming. I could feel the medicine working in my system, and even knew by my decline in mood when I would be due to have my next one! This had the added bonus of proving undoubtedly that my illness was hormonal in origin, and indeed could even be cured. The only thing the injection hadn't done was control my sporadic bleeding, which was so miserable and painful that I would often throw up.

On 29 November 2012 I received a full hysterectomy and oophorectomy (removal of ovaries), which was all done by key-hole surgery. When I woke up I couldn't have felt more relieved. I felt woozy and sleepy, but most of all I felt privileged that I had been able to receive this surgery, which was unavailable to so many. I was elated because not only had they been able to operate successfully, they had been able to do it without leaving a scar, and they had also rebuilt my entire pelvic cavity, so I was left with a beautiful designer vagina as well. The skill and professionalism of the surgical team had surpassed my expectations, and I felt so humble when they came to see me the next day. Apart from the fact that I had some blood loss on the table, the surgery couldn't have gone better. My research had also paid off, and it was during my recovery in hospital that I knew my life had changed forever. All of the tension was gone, all of the depression was gone and the feelings of madness had left me.

Within a few days I was home and initially there were no problems. By the following week, however, there was a serious bleed and I suddenly developed sepsis. When I was admitted to hospital, I was too ill to care, and the medical team had great problems trying to keep me alive throughout the night. The delirium was dreadful and I couldn't really tell what was going on. Poor Den and my mum were beside themselves, but as I recovered I began to feel quite philosophical about the whole thing. I knew deep down that the operation had transformed my life, so I considered the gamble and came to the conclusion that it was worth it. I also knew that the infection had definitely occurred because of my lowered immunity. Despite the seriousness of my condition I was allowed home for Christmas and I promised myself I would try harder to rescue my fragile physical health which had taken an enormous battering.

It took a long time to recover from such a big operation, some six months at least, and in the interim I was sometimes extremely frail. I simply couldn't do what I wanted to do, no matter how hard I tried, and I would often get extremely frustrated because I wanted to enjoy my new life and experience every 'balanced' moment. I would walk my little dog in the fields near our home, going a little further each time, and it was on one of these walks on a perishing winter's day that I knew the operation had definitely worked and my cure was here to stay.

I was normally far too cautious about the possibility of remission and was always waiting for a relapse, but as I looked around me I suddenly noticed how beautiful everything was. The sky was so big and everything looked so crisp, particularly the trees swaying gracefully in the breeze. I had never really noticed them before, and as I looked in the adjacent field there were horses grazing, which I had clearly overlooked on my previous strolls. It was like noticing everything for the first time, and my mind was able to 'look' rather than being lost to it all. I simply didn't have any of the negative and spiteful thoughts that had so damaged me in the past, and the patterns of my mind and mood were constant and unvarying. It made me wonder how I'd managed for so long the way I was, and I started to absorb just how sick I had been. I'd had no idea how bad I'd been until I experienced a life without symptoms. Looking back, I couldn't comprehend the magnitude of it all.

Even today I can recall this moment of clarity in great detail, and although it came at a price, it was something I felt so grateful for. I felt as though my whole body had given an enormous sigh of relief and I could start again and begin my recovery. Even though I had been robbed of much of my adult life, I felt like myself again, the person I was supposed to be, not the person that the illness had made me. I felt a sense of completeness; the search was over and the world really did look like a beautiful place.

Now over eight years later, my whole life has been transformed and, while I worry that there might be a relapse one day, I can't ignore the fact that I am still well. I don't suffer from any recurring ailments and I have a renewed energy which has allowed me to concentrate on writing this book. I am able to enjoy my children without the constant onslaught of depression and the endless cycle of despair. I am a better wife, a better mother and I have become passionate about raising awareness of the hormonal elements to this mood disorder. I am also fully aware that my recovery is completely dependent on the amazing scientists, doctors and health care professionals researching this condition. Without their professionalism and expertise, I really don't think I would be here.

PART 2

SELF-HELP FOR REPRODUCTIVE DEPRESSION

HORMONES AND REPRODUCTIVE ILLNESS

While writing this section of the book, I have kept the facts and terminology as simple and easy to understand as possible. I didn't want the text to be complicated or mystifying, because some of the books I've read on the subject have been far too complex, using medical terminology which can be overwhelming and almost reads like a foreign language. I have always been conscious that the hormonal elements of the illness can be confusing and difficult to grasp. The last thing anyone with a hormonal illness needs is to be overburdened with jargon that they can't realistically understand, particularly about the scientific elements involved in the body's production of hormones.

Keeping things simple is especially important for you, the reader, if you are unwell or have children to look after. I hope I have simplified the facts accordingly, and I also hope you can find valuable help in the diagnosis and management of your illness. With this in mind, the following chapters explain the reasons for hormonal depression, even though research is still fairly limited. I am forever hopeful that the work of both Professor Studd and the International Association for Premenstrual Disorders (IAPMD) will help to lessen the suffering for people with a hormonal illness and be practised in the mainstream.

My History

Even though everyone with reproductive depression has their own unique experience of it, the condition usually follows the timeline of starting in puberty, continuing throughout the reproductive years and then becoming climacteric (the point at which physical and emotional changes begin before the menopause), so that it peaks once the perimenopause (the phase before the menopause) begins. When one considers that these are the most critical and life-changing years of our lives, I think this makes reproductive depression a particularly brutal condition.

Timeline

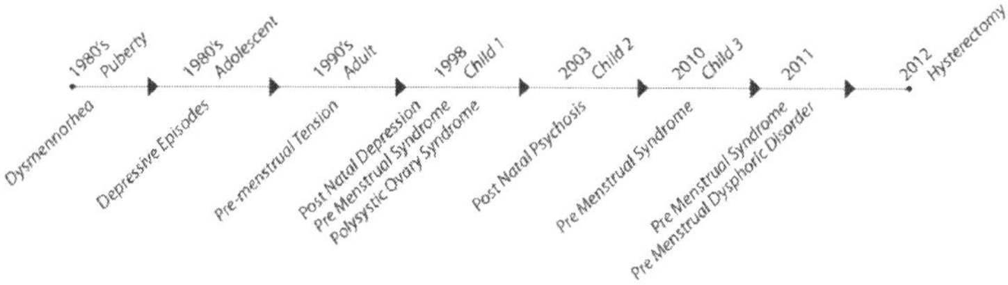

As you can see from the timeline above, the gradual progression of my own illness followed a very typical trajectory for reproductive depression. However, it is such a complicated and varied condition that the symptoms change dramatically every day, and in varying degrees from person to person. For me, I would have mostly physical issues during some months and then at other times my symptoms would be more mental. Sometimes there would be months where I would have a mixture of both.

After the birth of Billy I started reading, firstly at the library as at that particular point I had no access to the Internet, and after Freddie was born I read every available book and text I could get my hands on. By the time I'd had both children, I had cottoned on to the fact that there was something very wrong with me, but I was unable to accept that it was only a mental illness. Deep down, I knew that there was something biologically wrong. I had far too many physical symptoms which I simply couldn't ignore, and also my nursing experience was telling me that my immune system was somehow being seriously compromised. I was intrigued because I only ever experienced mental anguish after ovulation, rather than continuously. As I was only poorly for two weeks of every month, I was unable to accept the diagnoses of various psychiatrists and was adamant that there must be a physiological cause, rather than the 'bipolar illness' that they told me I had and yet which was mysteriously absent for the other fortnight of every month.

Reading other people's case studies made me acutely aware of the seriousness of the condition and I wanted to find a way to do it justice. By now I was in contact with other sufferers and was all too familiar with how dangerous and life-destroying the illness can be, and this spurred me on in my quest to get the details correct.

What Are Hormones?

Hormones, which are part of our endocrine system, are the chemicals inside our bodies which control all our physiological needs. We all have hormones and we simply couldn't function without them. Hormones work in a methodical and controlled way in a multi-functional, feedback system. One hormone will speak to another, and so they are known as chemical messengers. Put very simply, an endocrine gland (such as the ovary) will produce a hormone which then passes into the bloodstream and travels around the body until it arrives at a particular organ, which has the appropriate cells (known as receptor cells) so it can dock on to this organ and affect it in some way.

I am mostly going to talk about the reproductive hormones, although of course our bodies contain many other sorts of hormones as well. Together, these reproductive hormones control all aspects of the reproductive system. Some doctors refer to a group of hormones that work together like this as a hormonal orchestra.

For the purposes of this book, we are concerned with four sex hormones and their role in the female reproductive system.

Oestrogen This is a steroid hormone secreted mainly by the ovaries, although the adrenal cortex and placenta also secrete small amounts. Between puberty and the menopause, oestrogen helps to repair the inner lining (endometrium) of the womb following menstruation, ready for possible fertilization of an egg and subsequent pregnancy.

Progesterone This is a steroid hormone secreted by the ovaries, and also by the placenta during pregnancy to keep the foetus safely in the uterus. From puberty to the menopause, progesterone works with oestrogen to enrich the inner lining (the endometrium) of the womb to prepare it for pregnancy. The adrenal glands (one sits above each kidney) also secrete small amounts of progesterone.

FSH Its full name is follicle-stimulating hormone. It is synthesized and released by the anterior pituitary gland in the brain to stimulate the development of new follicles on the ovary each month.

LH LH stands for luteinising hormone, and it is synthesized and released by the anterior pituitary gland to stimulate ovulation and the formation of the corpus luteum (the tissue in the ovary that forms after ovulation and that secretes progesterone).

The Menstrual Cycle

As you can see from this graph, the menstrual cycle has pronounced hormonal peaks and troughs each month. The four hormones involved work together to enable us to menstruate and become pregnant. Their work begins at puberty and gradually tails off as we age, leading us into menopause.

Menstrual hormone variations during the menstrual cycle

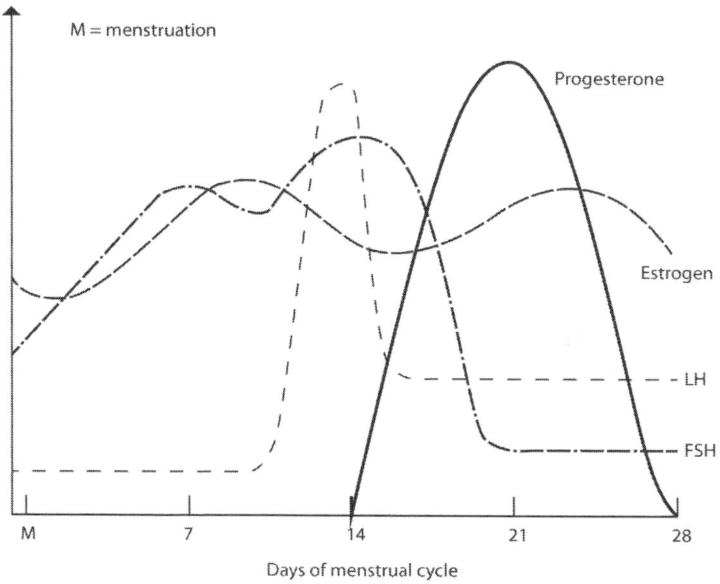

Each hormone plays a valuable part in this process and has an essential role, at an essential time. In particular, progesterone and oestrogen seem to be the most dominant, but others are also very active showing a whole host of fluctuations. Surprisingly testosterone is also present in females and is responsible for sex drive, muscle growth, bone density and body fat distribution.

Here is a brief description of how our hormones interact with each other every month. A new cycle begins at the end of menstruation, when levels of progesterone and oestrogen are low. Here's how it works.

1. FSH is secreted because of the drop in progesterone in the previous cycle. As its name suggests, FSH enables the new follicle on the ovary to develop into a mature egg. The levels of FSH continue to rise, triggering an increase in the production of oestrogen.
2. The oestrogen secreted from the ovaries starts to repair the lining of the uterus. As the levels of oestrogen rise, they switch off the FSH secretion and stimulate the production of LH (at about day 12, reaching a peak at day 14). Oestrogen is the main influence in the follicular phase – the first fourteen days of the menstrual cycle (on average) and which end with ovulation.
3. The LH causes ovulation and the development of the corpus luteum on the surface of the ovary. This is the luteal phase of the cycle, and it lasts for the last fourteen days of the cycle (on average). The corpus luteum begins to produce progesterone.
4. The progesterone secreted by the corpus luteum shuts down the production of FSH and LH, enriches the endometrium, keeps it in place and prevents any uterine contractions in case the egg that has been released embeds itself in the endometrium and starts to develop.
5. What happens next depends on whether the egg has been fertilized. If it has, the egg implants itself in the nutrient-rich lining of the endometrium and pregnancy begins. If no fertilization has taken place, the egg starts to die, the corpus luteum begins to break down, the progesterone levels drop and, as a result, the endometrium is shed and uterine contractions occur during menstruation. At the end of menstruation, the whole cycle starts again.

What Happens When Things Go Wrong

As you can see, this is a complex system of hormonal interplay, but what happens if it doesn't work correctly? What if there is an imbalance or a genetic fault that allows that system to be compromised? What if we damage this fragile system with our lifestyles or with the synthetic hormones that are often used in birth control? What happens to our whole mind–body system if we neglect the health of our hormones? What if we are particularly sensitive to these monthly changes and all that they entail?

If our hormonal system is damaged for some reason, not only does our mind suffer but our body will too. This results in a type of chemical chaos where one hormone can't guide another in the way it should, creating a long-term imbalance and a cycle of mental and physical ill health. The endocrine system and the parasympathetic nervous system (our body's soothing mechanism, which works in tandem with the sympathetic nervous system) are so interlinked that one can't possibly work efficiently without the other, and so an imbalance in one creates a huge biological problem that also results in physical trauma and mental difficulties. These can range from anxiety and depression to sexual difficulties and immunosuppression. In other words, you will become ill in various and multiple ways until that hormonal imbalance is corrected, or at least treated.

Another example of the problems that can develop when the hormonal system isn't working properly is Type 1 diabetes. My husband has this because his body does not and cannot produce insulin, which is a hormone produced by the pancreas to regulate the levels of glucose in the blood. His treatment for Type 1 diabetes is to inject himself with insulin every day, otherwise he will firstly get ill and then he will die. Replacing a hormone in this way sounds so simple, doesn't it? And yet it isn't, because if you throw another scenario into the hormone equation, such as hunger or a stressful situation, the hormones will need balancing again. It's the same if you use synthetic hormones, such as the contraceptive pill – the natural elements of the body are thrown out of sync, and that can disrupt the hormonal pathways. For some people this can have a critical and damaging effect on their physical health, followed by a catastrophic impact on their state of mind.

What if you are much more sensitive than other people to the changes in your hormones and can really sense them? For example, you might be able to tell immediately when you're ovulating, as this is another hormonal change. Or maybe you have known when you've become pregnant and can feel the mental and physical transitions, even though the pregnancy is at a very early stage. Most of us have heard someone say that they had a strong 'feeling' that they were pregnant, and that is exactly what I am trying to describe, the sense that a change has happened within our bodies. It is this so-called 'sensitivity' that can cause havoc for anyone who is so strongly affected by the subtle hormonal changes in their body each month that they become severely ill. This can be irrespective of the amount of hormones they are producing, and is most likely caused by the body's reaction to them.

As you read on you will see what can happen when you are so sensitive to your hormonal changes that they can radically change all of your bodily systems, making you ill, both mentally and physically. I have even heard of people experiencing a type of allergic reaction as soon as they ovulate. For others, the change in their brain chemistry is so profound that it 'mimics' mental illness, leading to what can be a life-long battle with depression, anxiety and ill health.

Now we are going to look at the different stages of the female reproductive cycle and how they can affect us.

Puberty

This is when hormonal upheaval is paramount. Puberty is the beginning of our sexual maturation, when we begin to develop secondary sexual characteristics. Boys' voices start to break and girls begin to grow breasts and also begin menstruating. It can be a turbulent time emotionally.

If you develop a hormonal illness at some point in your life, it's quite likely that you will have had some problems with depression and ill health during puberty, although sadly this correlation is not widely understood. Some teenage girls suffer from very heavy and painful periods (dysmenorrhea) while others have an absence of periods (amenorrhoea) or menstrual irregularities. The symptoms can affect their education and also their relationships with family and friends. There can be cycles of food cravings and depression, along with behavioural disturbances and even addictions. Hormonal imbalances during puberty can also lead to self-harm and suicide attempts, at a time in our lives when we are all most vulnerable.

Teenagers tend to eat sporadically and sometimes they have nutritional deficiencies which can have an added detrimental effect on their mood swings. Quite often a pubescent teenager will consult their doctor about these problems and will be given the contraceptive pill to help manage their symptoms. Sometimes the teenager will be regarded as being over-dramatic or attention-seeking but, mostly, their distress will be thought of as normal teenage angst and rarely picked up on.

In the first section of this book I described how my problems began during puberty but were simply overlooked. Even in my teens I was showing signs of severe depression and suicidal thoughts. I also had menstrual difficulties which disrupted my life so much that I asked for medical intervention. My relationship with alcohol, the promiscuity and obvious despair were already dominant but were dismissed as signs of depression. I'm hoping that this lack of understanding of the effects of hormonal illnesses will change in the future and anyone seeking professional help will, at the very least, be asked if there is a pattern between their low mood and their menstrual cycle. This can be monitored more closely by keeping a simple menstrual chart (see below) which will clearly show the timing and correlation of the mental and physical symptoms each month.

If you have never filled in a menstrual chart before, I am sure that you'll find it really helpful and possibly even illuminating. Once you have confirmed that your illness is cyclical, because you have charted the days or weeks when it's at its worst and the times when you don't notice it, you will be able to record more symptoms and whether they are physical, mental or both. Finding a pattern in your symptoms can be immensely empowering, and is often described as a 'light bulb moment'. Once you have established that you have a hormonal sensitivity to your own cycle, you can then decide on the appropriate treatment and medical intervention. You know what you are dealing with – it's no longer a mystery.

Menstrual Diary

	JAN	FEB	MAR	APR	MAY	JUN	JUL	AUG	SEP	OCT	NOV	DEC
1												
2												
3												
4												
5												
6												
7												
8												
9												
10												
11												
12												
13												
14												
15												
16												
17												
18												
19												
20												
21												
22												
23												
24												
25												
26												
27												
28												
29												
30												
31												

https://www.pms.org.uk/support/menstrual-diary/

The menstrual chart is the most valuable piece of information for anyone who wants to keep a detailed log of their symptoms and, more importantly, the time of the month when they occur.

If you keep a menstrual chart it will tell any doctor or other medical professional how often you are menstruating, and the symptoms, whether physical or mental, that occur during your cycle, such as before menstruation. Tracking the various ailments you have each month, and exactly when they happen, will reveal a regular and consistent pattern. You might have headaches which obviously you would mark on the chart with 'H', or depression and irritability which you would mark accordingly with 'D' and 'I' respectively, as you can see I have done with mine. In fact, you could include any type of symptom which you feel has become repetitive and troublesome. This will give you further insight into your cyclical illness.

By the time you have three months' worth of charts you should see a pattern emerging and you will gradually notice that you are indeed becoming ill at specific times each month. These illnesses can vary tremendously from person to person. For example, for years I have had bouts of shingles which, as you'll know if you've ever had them yourself, are painful and debilitating. A friend of mine pointed out, quite by chance, that I would have a flare-up at the same time every month – something that even I hadn't realized until she mentioned it. She, too, had hormonal problems and every month without fail would develop rhinitis, an uncomfortable allergy-type illness which would leave her snuffling like a hedgehog, unable to breathe. She also had severe mouth ulcers and burning mouth syndrome, which is incredibly painful. These symptoms would flare up just before each period, yet it was several months before the penny dropped and we both realized that she had the same illness as I did. It seems that if you have a slight illness or affliction, even something as simple as a bad back, it will show itself when you are premenstrual and will regularly cause you problems.

Another example of this is the terrifying nightmares and sleep paralysis I had, which would start as soon as I ovulated and which had plagued me throughout my menstrual history. One particular gynaecologist asked me how I knew when I was ovulating, and the simple answer was that my dreams would change and become far more hostile and menacing. The only reason I knew this was because I was keeping a menstrual chart and could see the correlation between the nightmares and ovulation for myself. So, for your own sake, and for the complete management of your health, keep a menstrual chart! You will soon see the pattern and this will enable you to take action. Once you have realized the significance and the timing of your symptoms, you have the proof you need when talking to any health care professionals. This means they can't fob you off or dismiss your symptoms, because you have the proof in front of you. You can manage the illness with multiple therapies, thereby reducing your symptoms dramatically and giving yourself the chance to lead a normal life. The only reason I have been able to achieve this myself is because I have kept and recognized the value of the menstrual chart.

Menstrual Diary Example

	JAN	FEB	MAR	APR	MAY	JUN	JUL	AUG	SEP	OCT	NOV	DEC
1				M		M	MH	M				
2				M		M	MH	M			M	M
3				M		M	MH	M	M		M	M
4				M	M		M	M	M		M	M
5			M	M			M		M		M	M
6			M	M	M		M		M		M	M
7			M	IDM	M		M		M		M	M
8				M	M		M				M	M
9				M	M	ID	M				M	M
10				M	M	ID	M				M	M
11				M	M						M	M
12				M	M	IDM					M	
13			IDB		M	IDM					M	
14			IDB	H	M	M					M	
15			IDB	IDH	M	M		ID		M	M	
Prozac Started → 16			B	IDH		M		ID		M		
17			B	ID				ID		M		
18			DB	ID				ID		M		
19			M	ID	IDB		M	ID		M		
20			IDM		IDB	M		M	M	M		
21			IDM	ID	M	M		M	M			M
22			IDM	ID	M	M		M	M			
23			IDM	IDM		M		M	M			
24				IDM		M		M	M			
25				M		M		M	M			
26				M		M		M	M			
27			ID	M								
28				IDM	IDB							
29			ID	HM			M					
30			IDB	IDM	IDB		M					
31			M		M		M					

M = Menstruation D = Depression B = Breast tenderness
H = Headache I = Irritability

I started this menstrual chart in 1999, which was the year after Freddie was born. You can see how often I was bleeding and the correlation between my depression and menstrual cycle. Once I started to use Prozac and natural progesterone, the depression and irritability gradually tailed off and, although I was still bleeding, the symptoms had lessened. By September of the same year, and with natural hormone intervention, I was gradually improving.

If you don't want to keep a physical chart, there are now various apps that can monitor both the timing of your symptoms and when they occur. These are available to download and have often been designed by sufferers and advocates of hormonal illness. These tracking devises can be a must-have in your emotional tool kit.

Here is a list of the apps that are most popular at the time of writing. I've given each one a rating of between three and five stars.

- Clue Period Tracker, Ovulation & Cycle Calendar *****
  Clue has tracking options related to literally everything in your body during your cycle. It seems to be the simplest one to use. Their website is at https://helloclue.com
- Flo Health & Period Tracker ****
  Flo records ovulation and also turns the data into useful graphs that show exactly what your body is doing and when. Their website is at https://flo.health
- Me v PMDD – Symptom & Treatment Tracker ***
  This is an app created by a mum for her daughter with PMDD and is affiliated with the International Association of Premenstrual Disorders (IAPMD). Their website is https://www.mevpmdd.com
- Balance – Menopause Support ***
  Balance was created by Dr Louise Newson who is on the Surgical Menopause Committee also at IAPMD. The app

includes surgical menopause and menopausal symptoms. Their website is https://balance-app.com

Pregnancy

It goes without saying that your hormonal levels during pregnancy are extremely high in order to nourish your unborn baby – your body is performing a complex balancing act of supplying all the hormones needed to keep the placenta and uterus healthy throughout your pregnancy. I was very well during my second pregnancy and, considering my circumstances, was positively vibrant. My hair and skin were glowing and I seemed to give off a type of luminosity. One friend remarked that I had a good 'aura', and a feeling of complete calmness surrounded me.

When you're pregnant it's quite normal to have some emotional moments, thanks to your body's hormonal fluctuations as a result of the pregnancy. This is particularly true in the first and last trimester, but it's usually when the baby is born that the hormone levels plummet and the hormonal sensitivity kicks in. This can leave you feeling tearful and exhausted on around day three, which is normally when your milk comes in. Feelings of despair are quite common (and are often called the 'baby blues') as you have probably been running on adrenalin for a few days. Stitches as a result of perineal tears, difficulties in breastfeeding and an overwhelming stream of visitors can leave you feeling bewildered and utterly exhausted, just at the point when you are most in need of rest. All of these emotions are entirely normal as the transition into motherhood is completed but, even though having a baby is a miraculous and wonderful experience, this life-changing event can also be traumatic for any new parents. One minute you are on cloud nine, and the next you would sell your soul for some normality or a decent night's sleep. As a mother of three bouncing baby boys, I still say that childbirth takes everything from you as a human being – all of your strength and all of your resolve – even if you feel well.

If you are hormonally sensitive, the change post-partum is even more dramatic. The following chart shows the sudden drop in hormone levels immediately after giving birth. Notice the sudden and dramatic reduction in progesterone secretion when a baby is born at week 40. This is what our bodies are so sensitive to and which can create a type of 'shock', resulting in illness and severe depression. Oestrogen levels drop too, although that isn't shown in the diagram.

Levels of progesterone during the menstrual cycle and pregnancy

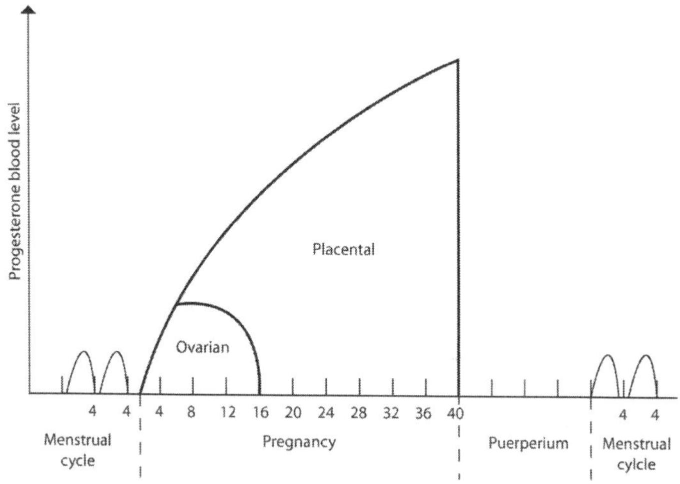

Post-natal Depression (PND)/Illness

Symptoms include:
Anxiety
Depression
Panic attacks
Chronic fatigue

Fibromyalgia
Depersonalization and feelings of unreality
Suicidal thoughts, whether passive or active
Failure to bond with the baby

For the purposes of this book, I have referred to what we used to call post-natal depression (PND) as post-natal illness. I have done this because the condition is responsible for so many physical symptoms, as well as mental disturbances, that I believe it should be known as an illness, rather than be categorized only as a depressive disorder.

For some women, having a baby poses no long-term health issues and their bodies cope really well, but for others 'the plummet' can be so drastic that their entire system experiences a type of collapse, plunging them into mental and physical crisis. What is the trigger? Once the pregnancy is over, and the baby and placenta have been delivered, the body has to return to normal function and 'switch on'. (Dr Katharina Dalton, who was an expert on PMS and hormonal imbalances, describes this as the menstrual clock.) For some women the switch can be traumatic, with a radical effect on all the body's systems in their entirety, encouraging the body to pump out adrenalin and the stress hormone cortisol. It seems that someone with a hormonal disease has abnormal surges of adrenalin and cortisol, although it has not yet been discovered why this is. This further unbalances the whole body, and also the mind, as the body desperately tries to maintain equilibrium. It is thought that the sudden drop in oestrogen and progesterone levels that occurs when the placenta is no longer present interferes with the serotonin and dopamine pathways in the brain. (Serotonin has many functions, which include regulating our behaviour and attention. Dopamine is a neurotransmitter that affects our experience of pleasure.) All of these chemicals play a vital role in our bodies, but if their balance is disturbed in any way this can have a drastic and sometimes devastating effect on the woman and her ability to care for her baby. Now the cycle of ill health begins, with far-reaching consequences for the new mother and sometimes also for the newborn infant. A history of depression means you are more likely to develop post-natal illness.

Post-natal illness is serious and devastating. It is not caused by the type of birth a woman had, her social standing or any obstetric factors. It will not go away of its own accord, either, so it requires urgent medical intervention and various professional therapies. It is also likely to be repeated in subsequent pregnancies, in which case it will require preventative measures to keep it at bay each time.

Surprisingly, post-natal depression can sometimes start with an episode of mania and excitability. Some people call this stage the 'baby pinks'. The euphoria and manic behaviour affect many women as a kind of upbeat prelude to the subsequent depression. Sometimes, however, post-natal depression will have the opposite effect, leaving the new mother drained and lethargic to the point where she refuses to get washed and dressed. Often the new mum will be hyper-anxious about the baby and won't let anyone else hold him or her. Alternatively, she might be indifferent to and detached from her newborn child. It's a disease with contradictory symptoms, and because every woman is an individual she will experience it in her own unique way.

The feelings of detachment that I had, known as depersonalization, or sometimes disassociation, when everything seems dreamlike and unreal, are extremely common. Some doctors believe it can be caused by severe anxiety and the flooding of adrenalin, and perhaps even cortisol (which is released in order to cope with all the stresses of being a new mother), through the body. These episodes of intense unreality are understandably terrifying for every new mother and the associated trauma can have long-lasting effects. Quite often this is when the woman will say that she is losing her mind or going crazy. Furthermore, we must not forget that all of this is happening after the birth of a child – an event that is supposed to be full of joy and hope – which is the saddest part of it all.

Although post-natal illness can and does have depressive symptoms, it is not to be confused with a normal depressive disorder. Ordinary depression can cause acute insomnia, however when I had reproductive depression I would feel an absolute compulsion to sleep, which lasted for many years. Some women I've talked to say that it's like having jetlag or even that they feel 'drugged up', which I now know to be called chronic fatigue syndrome. Others have big issues with insomnia, which can be debilitating and exhausting. As you can see, the symptoms can be very individual.

Post-natal depression is a very sneaky condition and one that can creep up without any warning. There are no rules about when it can strike, either – you might develop it several years after giving birth. The post-partum phase is so complex that it is often misunderstood. Quite often, it is confused with exhaustion, being in pain, lack of sleep, and the highly emotional transition into motherhood and the responsibilities that come with it. Because of these emotional reactions, sometimes you can have post-natal depression but you put it down to tiredness or exhaustion, or the trauma of birth. On the other hand, some women know they are ill but hide it because they are ashamed or are frightened about what will happen to them and their family if they are diagnosed with post-natal depression. I have spoken to some women who were so worried that their baby would be taken away from them that they kept their true feelings secret and struggled on without telling a soul. Many women are reluctant to speak out because of innate guilt and a fear of being judged. Having suffered from post-natal illness myself I can categorically say that it is one of the worst things anyone can endure and the potential suicide risk can lead to incomprehensible tragedy. Professor John Studd has an abundance of information on this topic on his website. The references below also offer more information and ongoing support.

Useful websites
Professor John Studd at https://www.studd.co.uk/postnataldepression.php
Association for Post Natal Illness at https://apni.org
PND Awareness and Support (PaNDAS) at https://pandasfoundation.org.uk

Post-natal Psychosis

Symptoms include:
Hallucinations
Delusions
Loss of reality
High mood (mania)
Confusion
Agitation
Restlessness
Sleep problems

This is the most serious of all the hormonal illnesses, normally resulting in hospital admission to a secure unit. You can shift very quickly from being a normal, healthy and competent mother to one who is extremely ill. Psychosis happens when you lose touch with reality, and the symptoms can vary widely. Normally there is a loss of maternal instinct, so you might be unable to care for your infant and any other children you might have. You might feel indifferent towards the baby to the point of being unable to bond with him or her at all, or you might become so paranoid and over-protective that you're afraid to let the baby out of your sight. There are usually delusions of some kind and/or feelings of unreality. There are sleep problems too, and many episodes of post-natal psychosis begin with nightmares and hallucinations.

Post-natal psychosis is so dangerous if it's left untreated that urgent medical attention is essential in order to protect the life of the baby and the mother. It is a medical emergency and is not something the mother will snap out of after a good night's sleep! Time is of the essence as a delay in treatment can hinder the chance of a swift recovery for the mother. If the mother is so ill that she cannot recognize the need for help, or has become so paranoid that she dare not entrust her baby's care to anyone other than herself, then her partner or someone else must act on her behalf urgently and summon the help that is so obviously needed, either by contacting her GP or midwife, or taking her to the nearest A&E unit. Sometimes the mother may be so ill that she needs to be treated in hospital, ideally in a Mother and Baby Unit (MBU), until she is better. The MBU enables the mother and baby to stay together while the mother receives psychiatric treatment.

Useful websites

Professor John Studd at https://www.studd.co.uk/postnatalpsychosis.php

Action on Postpartum Psychosis at https://www.app-network.org

Premenstrual Syndrome (PMS)

Symptoms include:

Depression and anxiety

Mood swings

Irritability

Agitation
Headaches
Breast tenderness
Acne
Food cravings

Although the terms are sometimes used interchangeably, premenstrual syndrome (PMS) is not another name for premenstrual tension (PMT). My understanding of PMT is that it is a milder version of PMS and it lasts for a shorter amount of time, with less severe symptoms. PMS is a cyclical illness that results in a collection of mental and physical conditions that are severe enough to need medical treatment every month. As with the other conditions discussed in this book, some of the symptoms caused by hormonal fluctuations (the so-called premenstrual tension or PMT) in any given month are perfectly normal. However, if you have PMS you will experience a gradual change of character each month, starting around the time of ovulation and getting worse until menstruation begins. The cyclical nature of the illness is the vital clue that leads to a successful diagnosis of PMS.

Between ovulation and menstruation you might have Jekyll and Hyde mood swings as well as profound exhaustion which makes you so tired that you have to spend a lot of time in bed. You might be intensely irritable and agitated, and may become so sensitive to certain noises that you can't bear to hear them. The medical name for this condition is misophonia (hatred of sound). Not surprisingly, these extreme mood swings, high levels of irritation and inability to tolerate certain sounds can wreak havoc in your relationships, whether they're with your partner, children, family, friends or colleagues. Everyone around you may feel that they're tiptoeing around on eggshells for most of the time, afraid of triggering another angry outburst for what seems to be no apparent reason. Their lives are turned upside down and so is yours. The terrible depression that can strike just before ovulation often results in more mood swings, as well as anxiety, panic attacks, aggression, severe irritability, swearing, tantrums, irrationality, crying, self-harm, suicidal thoughts and a total inability to cope. This will continue until your period arrives and you begin to feel better.

As well as these symptoms of mental illness, PMS can involve physical illnesses that crop up at the same point in the menstrual cycle each month, often resulting in repeated doctors' appointments, hospital admissions and days off work. For me, the symptoms included flu-like aches and pains, water retention, food cravings, headaches and migraines, breast tenderness, nymphomania, low blood sugar, acne, asthma, mouth ulcers, cold sores, urinary infections, palpitations, vertigo, burning mouth, shingles and exhaustion.

As you can see from the hormonal timeline I showed you at the start of this section of the book, my illness probably began with this syndrome, but as it was not diagnosed correctly it gradually evolved into post-natal illness and then psychosis. I know of some cases where PMS began with post-natal depression and progressed from there. Whichever way it starts, if you develop PMS it will always have a detrimental effect on your lifestyle and will always require some sort of medical intervention, as you have seen from my own experience.

Useful websites

National Association for Premenstrual Syndromes at https://www.pms.org.uk

Premenstrual Dysphoric Disorder (PMDD)

Symptoms include:

Depression and anxiety

Mood swings
Irritability
Agitation
Headaches
Breast tenderness
Fibromyalgia
Chronic fatigue
Acne
Food cravings
Self-harm
Suicide attempts
Disruption to family life
Disruption in the workplace
Violence and criminality

This is another cyclical condition that can make life a misery between ovulation and the start of your period. It is caused by your body's extreme sensitivity to the natural changes in oestrogen and progesterone that govern your menstrual cycle every month. Although PMDD is usually regarded as an endocrine disorder, meaning that hormones are the culprits, it can trigger a whole host of mental and physical symptoms that begin each month at ovulation and continue until menstruation begins. At its most extreme, you may only feel normal for a maximum of five days a month. One of the most notable symptoms of PMDD is the way it can completely disrupt your life. No wonder that friendships, marriages and other relationships can fracture or be destroyed when someone has PMDD.

As with the other hormonal illnesses I've described, the symptoms of PMDD are very varied, so your experience of it might be very different to that of someone else who has it. One of the symptoms that is hardest to manage is an all-consuming depression. I've spoken to people with PMDD who complain of 'near-death experiences' every month, making them continually at risk of violence to others and themselves, as well as self-harm and suicide. If you have PMDD at its worst, you'll feel unable to cope with almost anything life throws at you. You may cut off all social contact because you can't deal with it or you don't have the mental or physical energy for it. You might even find it difficult to be around friends because they simply don't understand how you're feeling. Added to this, your thoughts might be so scattered that you're continually forgetful, you seem unable to speak coherently or you can't concentrate on anything for long. You may also find you're acutely sensitive to noise and/or light, so going to a crowded pub or busy restaurant is the last thing you want. You just want to run away.

PMDD requires medical intervention by a competent endocrinologist or gynaecologist and will not get better without this help. The first step is to talk to your GP. Show them your menstrual charts for at least the past three months, so you have proof of the cyclical nature of your mental and physical symptoms, especially if you're finding it difficult to describe them or you're worried about not being taken seriously. If left untreated, PMDD can lead to hospital admissions, for both psychiatric and physical symptoms, at regular times each month and creates a cycle of utter misery both for you and for those around you. Prisons and psychiatric units across the world are full of inmates with PMDD, who quite often have been violent and criminal. It is by far the most persistent and troublesome form of reproductive depression.

Useful websites

International Association for Premenstrual Disorders at https://iapmd.org

Mind at https://www.mind.org.uk/media-a/2947/pmdd-2017.pdf

Premenstrual Exacerbation of an Underlying Disorder (PME)

Symptoms include:
Anxiety
Severe depression
Suicidal thoughts or actions
Alcoholism
Eating disorders
Violence and criminality

This illness is exactly what its name implies. If you already have a physical or mental health condition, it can be magnified or made worse when your hormonal levels fluctuate during the late luteal phase of your cycle. Your body's production of inflammatory proteins at this stage of the cycle can also trigger a disorder, whether it's physical or mental. Two examples of this are bipolar disorder and major depressive disorder, both of which will almost certainly worsen in the late luteal phase each month. Examples of physical problems that flare up in the second half of the menstrual cycle can be anything from arthritis to a debilitating physical illness such as Crohn's disease, colitis, epilepsy or asthma.

Trying to distinguish between PME and PMDD is extremely difficult because the symptoms can often overlap. One clue, however, is that with PME you will have some symptoms throughout your entire cycle but they will worsen during the premenstrual phase, whereas with PMDD the symptoms only appear post-ovulation and then improve once your period starts. In order to be certain, you need a thorough medical diagnosis. Of course, both conditions deserve treatment and understanding.

It may not be a case of having either PMDD or PME, because you might have both. The same is true of bipolar disorder and

PMS. As poor mental health can lead to more problems, I am no longer surprised when I hear of someone who has had one, two or even multiple diagnoses. In medical terms, this is known as having comorbidity.

As with the other reproductive illnesses discussed here, it's important to fill in menstrual charts for at least three months, so you can show the medical professionals you talk to how your condition affects you on a day-to-day basis. You will need to try any protocol you're using, such as SSRI or homeopathy, for three months before you see a result. Patience and persistence are key.

Useful websites

International Association for Premenstrual Disorders at https://iapmd.org/pmdd-v-pme

Menopause

Many women sail through the menopause with very few difficulties, while others have a host of problems ranging from depression and anxiety, to vaginal dryness and low libido.

Quite often I've seen the problematic side of menopause and many even refer to this time as their second puberty because it creates such hormonal upheaval. In terms of timing, it couldn't be more difficult, with many of us entering this climacteric phase at the same time as the onset of puberty for our own teenagers, and the decline of our own parents' health as well. This double whammy massively increases our stress levels, which in turn increases the problematic symptoms of reproductive depression.

If you consider that reproductive depression often follows the trajectory of post-natal depression, premenstrual depression and climacteric depression, and is often treated by having a hysterectomy, it's very easy to be caught out in the climacteric phase by the severity of the symptoms, in particular depression and anxiety. You might imagine that having a surgical menopause (hysterectomy, plus the removal of the ovaries and fallopian tubes) means no more hormonal difficulties, yet you might still have problems getting the balance of your HRT right, and you might even find that you don't absorb enough oestrogen through a patch that you wear or a gel that you apply to your skin.

One of the more serious episodes I had after my hysterectomy was when I was lulled into a false sense of security by having a patch in situ, despite it not giving me a high enough level of oestrogen to keep me well. I also massively underestimated the importance of add-back testosterone, which is vital for energy levels and sex drive.

Be prepared to monitor your condition consistently, even if you've had a hysterectomy or your ovaries removed. I seemed to have a decline in oestrogen after my surgical menopause in 2012, but also another dip during 2019 which had a catastrophic effect on my mental and physical health. I can only hazard a guess and say that this coincided with what would have been my natural menopause time, as my mother suffered similar issues at that age. Alternatively, it could have been that my oestrogen levels were so depleted – <19 pmol/l to be precise – that the mood crash was almost certainly inevitable.

Professor Studd has stated categorically that oestrogen levels should be between 200 pmol/l and 600pmol/l, so don't get caught out. For those of us who have PND, PMDD and PMS, anything less than 200pmol/l will probably have a negative outcome for us, and can even bring on a full-blown episode. I can't stress enough how important it is to have regular blood tests and to even keep a mood diary or chart to show the menopause clinic, should you need to.

If you are still having significant problems, the oestrogen and testosterone can be given via an implant which goes deeper under the skin and usually have an even better result for blood plasma levels.

Implants are convenient, especially if you have had a hysterectomy or have tried other therapies. They also have the added bonus of increasing your bone density, particularly of your lumbar spine, and they also increase your energy and libido. Regular checks that your implant is still working properly are paramount for your ongoing health, particularly if you have this particular disorder. Ask for regular check-ups, don't be fobbed off, and don't be lulled into a false sense of security.

How to Know When to Have a Hysterectomy

Although a hysterectomy may seem radical, for many of us it is the closest thing we currently have to a cure.

Often someone with hormonal illness will have exhausted all the other options available to them before they decide that a hysterectomy is the only answer. It's their last resort because they've run out of all the others. Obviously, it's a permanent solution, so it is often the choice of someone who has completed their own family. However, it can also be choice of someone who has decided that their appalling symptoms are too hard to live with and that bearing their own children is never going to be an option. This is often through fear of passing on their illness to their children – we now know that reproductive depression can and does often run in families. They might also feel profoundly anxious about how to cope with both the symptoms of the illness and the realities of child-rearing. All of this is perfectly understandable. There are no rights and wrongs about the decision to have major surgery.

If you do decide to take this route, you need to know that you can't have only your uterus removed. A hysterectomy for someone with a hormonal illness must be accompanied by the removal of both ovaries and both fallopian tubes. This is known as a bilateral salpingo-oophorectomy (BSO) and it will stop all symptoms. Professor Studd always advocates the use of add-back

HRT to protect the heart and bones, with both oestrogen and testosterone given for optimal health.

BSO is a major operation and therefore it isn't without risk. So how do you know when surgery is worth taking that risk? While writing this I asked in the many forums I belong to what was the final straw for someone before they decided to have BSO. Quite often people replied that they had several reasons, with many saying that they couldn't stand living with so many different symptoms any longer. Many of them told me that they simply knew when the time had come and often added that the surgery has transformed their lives. Even so, if you are considering such a radical step you must weigh up the risks before going under the knife. Ask yourself the following questions to help you decide.

- Have you have exhausted the trajectory in the NICE guidelines for PMS?
- Are you in extreme physical pain which is unmanageable and doesn't respond to any pain relief, whether it's conventional or a form of complementary medicine?
- Do you have chronic fatigue and/or fibromyalgia?
- Do you have lowered immunity, with recurrent infections or illnesses?
- Are you severely anaemic because of heavy periods and disease pathology?
- Are you self-harming in any way or do you have issues with addiction?
- Are you struggling to keep a good work–life balance?
- Has your condition led to marital and/or family problems?
- Are your symptoms causing you to be violent or involved in criminal activity?
- Lastly, and most importantly, do you have suicidal thoughts and have you ever attempted suicide?

Even if you answer 'yes' to several of these questions, you still need to consider your next step very carefully. It is vital to try several of the less invasive treatment options (this includes complementary medicine if it appeals to you) before considering surgery. As I've said before, it's essential to track your symptoms because that will validate what you are saying about your condition and enable your GP or consultant to see how you are affected by hormonal illness each month. You should also do your best to educate yourself as much as possible about BSO and weigh up the pros and cons before reaching a decision about what to do next.

Alice's Story

'It's called PMDD,' my GP told me as I sat, broken, in his office. I always knew there was something different about the way I was and how I reacted. I often experienced emotions more strongly than my friends, but I never understood why my mood would flip overnight. This was the third doctor's office I had sat in, trying to explain my symptoms, but this time was different, I was being heard and believed.

Being a midwife had its own tragic irony for me because my PMDD symptoms were so severe that I was considered treatment-resistant. The mask that I would have to wear when at work was so tight and restrictive that it started to fuse with my face and my real self was pushed deeper and deeper until I was unrecognizable. I became so skilled at hiding my true pain when I wore my uniform that nobody could see my illness for what it was.

I was a high-functioning PMDD sufferer and managed to hold down a job, and even get a promotion within midwifery. I filled my days with work and study, and my evenings with one hobby after another, never feeling satisfied and never feeling fulfilled.

I was so consumed with appearing normal and being the perfect midwife, the perfect friend, daughter and wife that when my PMDD symptoms arrived they knocked me sideways and I would often find myself sitting in the corner of a dark room crying so hard that my head would physically hurt.

The pain came gushing out during the late luteal phase of my cycle, hitting hardest on day 21. This would be my flashpoint that triggered a torrent of rage, depression, suicidal thoughts and fear. Yet day after day I would slip on my uniform, put on the mask and go to work. I would walk the halls of the maternity unit with a smile on my face even though I was screaming inside.

Having a reproductive health disorder while supporting countless women became unbearable. Being treatment-resistant meant that my only hope of sanity was to suppress the monthly cycle and undergo a chemical menopause.

Growing up I had a strong maternal instinct. I dreamt of raising a large family, with a dog and a white picket fence. PMDD was robbing me of this chance and I watched it get stripped away piece by piece. Every day I would take medication to prevent ovulation and try to keep myself alive, but cruelly my body's natural instinct was to become a mother and was so strong it would put up a fight, one that I always lost.

In 2016 I had reached the end of my journey to become a mother and booked my surgery for a hysterectomy and removal of my ovaries. My last day at work before the operation was heartbreaking. As I delivered my last baby of the shift into the arms of his new parents, I cried with them. I would never know that feeling of pure joy that exists in the moments after a birth, where the world stops spinning and all that there is is that moment frozen in time.

Walking into the operating theatre were the hardest steps I had ever taken, but I had no other options. PMDD was trying to kill me, I didn't want to pass it down to my child and so I let go of my dream of being a mother.

I would love to say that my recovery was easy, uncomplicated and that my PMDD had disappeared. Technically, yes, it had, I no longer had a menstrual cycle. Unfortunately it was never that easy.

Going back into clinical midwifery was harder than I ever could have imagined. My PMDD mask was gone but it was replaced with another, a raw and unexpected grief. I was grieving the loss of potential motherhood and doubted myself both as a woman and a midwife.

The word 'midwife' comes from the old English term 'with woman'. Could I truly call myself a midwife when I doubted my own womanhood? How could I be that source of comfort and stability when I was not there for myself? I retreated into a dark depression and I just couldn't find my way out.

After yet another suicide attempt, I finally reached out for professional help and was also diagnosed with depression and PTSD. Working as a midwife was no longer a realistic option for me. The pain was too raw and with every new birth, every new mother, the pain was ripped open.

It was two years after my surgery that I finally found some hope. I realized that I could use my personal experience of PMDD and my professional knowledge to give back to the PMDD community. As a midwife, being 'with woman' need not be restricted to the short nine months of a woman's life when she bears children. Reproductive health means so much more than that. My path was laid out for me.

With the unconditional love of my wife Sarah, we founded a not-for-profit organization to empower women and people assigned female at birth to become advocates for their own reproductive health. PMDD and Me was an idea that came to me suddenly on a bus one day. Lingering at the back of my mind was the solution to my grief but I had been so consumed with it that I had forgotten the bigger picture.

As a health care professional I was trained to recognize ante-natal and post-natal depression and was skilled in recognizing personality disorders, depression and anxiety. But never in all my training had I heard the term PMDD. If I as a midwife couldn't identify my own reproductive health disorder, how could anyone else do the same?

In two short years Sarah and I have channelled our energy into PMDD and Me. I have taken something that quite literally was killing me and turned it into something truly beautiful. We believe in the fundamental right to reproductive health and are beginning to make a difference.

In 2019 we hosted the first conference for people with PMDD in the UK and reached people in over twenty countries across six continents. We now run regular webinars and forums for experts to deliver evidence-based teaching and have an outreach program based in Kenya. We plan to take our teaching into schools and universities.

Our goal for the future is to embed reproductive health into the national curriculum. No longer can it be acceptable to ignore the credible scientific link between menstrual cycles and psychology. We must begin these conversations with our children today and break the cycle of menstrual shame.

Midwives and nurses must be taught about PMDD and other reproductive illnesses in their training and know how to recognize the obvious symptoms that sadly can take twelve years to diagnose.

My future may not be the one I had dreamed about years ago, but I wouldn't change it for anything. I may no longer be a midwife in the traditional sense but I believe I am now more 'with woman' than ever before. Having a condition like PMDD has made me into the person that I am today and has opened new doors and opportunities. I have taken my diagnosis and turned it into something wonderful.

For that I will be forever grateful.

Alice Girling is a reproductive health specialist, higher education lecturer and co-founder of PMDD and Me Community Interest Company. For over twenty years Alice suffered from treatment-resistant PMDD, which presented itself from puberty, before having a hysterectomy and removal of her ovaries in 2016. She now works to empower advocacy and raise awareness of reproductive health through her not-for-profit organization that she has founded with her wife, Sarah

CAUSES

In this section of the book I'm going to discuss the causes of reproductive disease. You'll find some of the solutions in the following section on treatments.

Genetics

For some time now, Harvard University in the US and the National Institute of Health, Maryland, have been conducting ongoing research into the causes of reproductive depression. They had a breakthrough in 2007 when they finally managed to isolate the gene responsible. It is called Catechol-O-methyltransferase or COMT, and is the first significant genetic finding in this so-called reproductive depression. Normally, COMT is involved in the functioning of neurotransmitters including dopamine, but when it is damaged it can send your mood regulation haywire. This then has a catastrophic effect on your state of mind as you move into the late luteal phase of your cycle each month. Reproductive depression can be hereditary and has no link to your personal circumstances, as this latest finding proves. Unfortunately, some factors can make the symptoms even worse and increase the possibility of yet more complications, so in the end reproductive depression becomes a progressive illness.

One thing that is certain is that the gene findings clarify that reproductive depression is a biological illness with biological manifestations. Methylenetetrahydrofolate reductase (MTHFR), which is a regulatory enzyme produced in the body, also has genetic variations which can trigger all sorts of mental health disorders. If you are unlucky enough to have two gene variants, as I have, then you will undoubtedly have health issues of varying degrees. Quite often these gene variants can lie dormant for many years but that can change at any time – this is known as epigenetics.

If you want to know more, and get your own genetic report, 23andMe is a company that is collecting data on gene expression. If you send them a sample of your saliva they'll produce a report that goes into your genetic inheritance and lists the health conditions that are associated with your DNA. This information can help you to make decisions about many aspects of your health, including diet and exercise, enabling you to manage your illness regardless of its origin.

Useful websites

23andMe at https://www.23andme.com/en-gb/

Stress

Stress can affect any of us at any time, and our hectic lives often make us feel increasingly pressured and anxious. As soon as we begin to feel stressed or worried, our bodies are immediately flooded with cortisol and adrenalin, two stress hormones that are designed to put us into the fight or flight response. Working together, they increase our heart rate, speed up our breathing and send energy to our muscles, so we can either run away from danger or stand our ground and fight. For our far-off ancestors, it was exactly what they needed when facing a wild beast. However, our bodies can't tell the difference between a hungry animal that wants to eat us and everyday tensions, such as a frustrating traffic jam, scary credit card bill or yet another argument with a member of the family. The physiological effects are the same – our body activates our sympathetic nervous system and adrenocortical system, with our hypothalamus and pituitary glands both secreting hormones to help us cope with whatever danger we are facing. If we need to take physical action we can immediately put those hormones to good use – we've all heard stories of people who were suddenly capable of amazing physical feats in a crisis, such as a parent somehow finding the strength to lift a car off their injured child, thanks to the surge of stress hormones in their body. However, if we're dealing with mental or emotional stress instead, those hormones will start to cause chemical chaos inside us because we have no way of burning them off. This sort of stress can have a very serious effect on the human immune system, and can even lower the number of white blood cells that our bodies need to fight infections. No wonder we can go down with a bad cold or some other illness after a period of stress.

If you have reproductive depression, persistent or chronic stress will only worsen your symptoms because of the cascade of chemicals it can trigger. It's as though your body's stress response is permanently switched on. This interferes with your body's hormone responses, making you increasingly susceptible to infections and illnesses, and has the potential to cause insulin resistance, brain fog and even damage to your body's ability to metabolize sex hormones.

Poor Nutrition

Did you know that you can eat three meals a day but still have poor nutrition? It happens when the food you eat doesn't contain what your body needs, such as enough vitamins, minerals, trace elements and essential fatty acids (EFA). Poor nutrition can lead to many mental and physical ailments, including hormonal imbalances. Regularly eating too many processed foods, toxins and sugar will take its toll on your hormones, and can even lead to digestive problems. A poor diet, especially if it's laden with sugar, can also cause insulin resistance which can lead to diabetes.

If you aren't eating a decent diet – which really means cooking your meals from scratch whenever possible rather than taking them out of a packet and putting them in the microwave – you will start to have food cravings. These are messages from your body, telling you what it wants you to eat. Unfortunately, these messages can get confused with cravings for the foods that aren't good for you. For instance, eating too much sugar can lead to a negative cycle of feeling tired and hungry, and satisfying it with something sweet which causes a spike in your blood sugar, followed by a slump in energy once your body has worked hard to get rid of the excess blood sugar, making you reach for another sugary snack to give you another boost of energy. And so it goes on! Hunger can lead to all sorts of adverse symptoms and might even wake you up at night, which is when your blood sugar levels often drop. These fluctuating levels of blood sugar can trigger the release of adrenalin which, as I've already explained, is a stress hormone that can cause its own set of physical problems.

Stimulants and Chemicals

If you have a hormonal illness, any sort of stimulant is going to aggravate it by triggering your stress hormones and disturbing your brain chemistry. Stimulants include caffeine, nicotine, alcohol and all narcotics. Narcotics in particular will interfere with your body's production of serotonin, the so-called feel good neurotransmitter.

Too many stimulants can leave you feeling jazzed up for hours afterwards. They can even interfere with your sleep patterns and lead to insomnia, as you'll know if you've ever drunk too many cups of coffee late at night. This is problematic for three reasons. Not only will you feel tired the next day, making you more likely to reach for food and drink that will wake you up (and which therefore contain yet more stimulants), but your body won't have had enough time overnight to carry out its vital repair work while you were asleep. And, if you have a hormonal illness, chronic insomnia can make things worse. That's because it's your hormones that regulate your sleep, with progesterone, oestrogen and testosterone all playing vital roles. Disturbed hormones can mean disturbed sleep patterns.

As well as the chemicals we are consuming in our food and inhaling in polluted environments, there are many synthetic chemicals around us which are known 'hormone disruptors'. These include synthetic hormones such as the contraceptive pill in all its forms, pesticides, plastic compounds and industrial elements, all of which further damage our already fragile hormonal system. Even the moisturisers and cosmetics we use can contain hormone disruptors, such as parabens, so it pays to read the ingredients labels and to choose products that are as free from all synthetic chemicals as possible. At its worst, this daily chemical onslaught from so many different products can cause learning disabilities, cognitive developmental issues and thyroid problems. Some hormone disruptors are now being removed from the market because scientists and regulators are recognizing and identifying their adverse effects on us.

Something else to consider, and which may not have immediately occurred to you, is the type of sanitary protection you use. Whether it's tampons, sanitary pads or a combination of both, do your best to buy the ones made from organic materials. Ordinary tampons and pads may contain dioxins and other toxins that result from the process of bleaching cotton to make it white. Because you wear the pads next to your skin, or tampons inserted in your vagina, these toxins will be in close contact with your mucous membranes. If you currently use tampons, you could consider switching to pads to see if they improve your symptoms.

Intolerances

Some food intolerances are known to interfere with our hormones and can even exacerbate the symptoms of hormonal illness. If you have a food intolerance it means that you have some sort of adverse reaction whenever you eat that food. This isn't the same as having a food allergy, which is when you are so allergic to a particular food, such as nuts, that your life might be in danger if you eat it.

Food intolerances include dairy, wheat and sugar, all of which can further unbalance us by creating a cycle of bingeing, mood swings, irritability and even poor memory. Although it sounds counterintuitive, if you are intolerant of a food you can end up craving it, so you become addicted to it and intolerant of it at the same time. Food intolerances can even be responsible for digestive problems, such as bloating or indigestion, which in turn can aggravate an already overloaded stress system. Research has discovered that gastrointestinal inflammation, which is one of the most frequent symptoms of a food intolerance, accompanies many mental health conditions. Obviously, if you have a food allergy you will know the importance of avoiding that food at all costs, but if you have a history of seasonal allergies, such as hay fever, you can't take the same avoiding action. These sorts of allergies can be responsible for many symptoms affecting the central nervous system and even the brain itself, and can lead to mood disorders.

If you have reproductive depression you will have a complete intolerance to progesterone or at least to progestin (the synthetic form of progesterone). Recent research into hormonal contraceptives has found a clear link between them and depression and anxiety, which is no big surprise when you consider that most contraceptives are full of synthetic progesterone. Deciding which form of contraceptive to use can be a difficult choice when you have a hormonal illness, unless you are happy to use a simple barrier method such as condoms or a diaphragm (known as a Dutch cap in the US), or to trust the rhythm method. I suggest discussing it with your GP or other health care professional, as well as your partner.

Trauma

Childhood trauma is one of the most significant reasons for depression later in life. Numerous studies have shown a hormonal component to trauma: put simply, the system that controls your body's reaction to stress is called the HPA axis (so-named because it involves a connection between the hypothalamus, pituitary gland and the adrenal glands). When you are caught up in a long-term stressful situation, your HPS axis becomes damaged and, to put it simply, gets jammed in the 'on' position. Your adrenal glands become exhausted, resulting in mood swings and low energy, among other problems.

Difficult experiences in early life, such as sexual trauma, emotional abuse or neglect, will significantly increase your body's tendency to over-react to what it considers to be any stressful situation. This often means that someone who is clinically depressed can be resistant to conventional pharmaceutical treatment and might face a lifetime of ill health as a result.

The problem with reproductive depression is that it often leads to further problems. Having any clinical illness can be so traumatic that it eventually triggers Complex Post-traumatic Stress Disorder (CPTSD). So a trauma from childhood, whatever that may be, can deregulate your stress response to such a degree that you now have two or even three more diagnoses.

The presence of multiple disorders is known as comorbidity and is far more common than you might think, with conditions which can and do overlap. A massive 51% of patients with psychiatric conditions have another ongoing health issue which makes treatment options more difficult to determine. Bipolar disorder, for example, has very similar symptoms to PMDD. Comorbidity also complicates the therapy options because the health care professional in charge of the case has to work out which was the primary condition.

Trauma can also lead to problems with addictions, and current research aims to tackle and highlight this. The onset of Post-traumatic Stress Disorder can often lead to some form of substance abuse, which can be self-soothing behaviour, and quite often when treating this it is important to understand the initial trauma and when it happened. Someone who experiences trauma in adolescence will often begin to have difficulties with their reproductive cycle and pubescent hormonal surges. Younger children who have experienced severe and prolonged trauma will often go on to have a multitude of health conditions throughout their entire lives. Almost certainly they have remained in fight or flight mode, which can lead to feelings of unreality or disassociation as adrenalin and cortisol continue to flood their system.

Our physical health is also powerfully affected by trauma, and can lead to innumerable illnesses, particularly those with a hormonal basis. Being stuck on high alert or experiencing flashbacks and/or nightmares can destabilize both our physical and emotional responses for many years afterwards. Exposure to serious trauma can lead to suicidal thoughts and, sadly, suicide.

Endogenous

Endogenous' is a term with several medical meanings, but when used in a psychiatric context it means that there don't appear to be any external reasons for the patient's condition. In other words, being diagnosed with endogenous reproductive depression means that no one knows what caused it.

This can make life rather frustrating if you are searching for a reason for your depression, because you can't identify any particular trigger. Many people who have had an emotional illness often say that they had wonderful childhoods with no trauma, or they are happily married and are astonished when they become ill.

By nature we automatically assume that there must have been an event or a catastrophe to warrant such a decline in emotional and physical health. Quite often there is no such event (except for the fluctuations in hormones) which was serious enough to trigger someone's heightened sensitivity and vulnerability. The cause of their condition remains a mystery. However, that doesn't mean it is any less real or genuine.

The Full Picture

Having looked at the genetic variations, the hormone disruptors and the stressful elements of life, we can clearly see how a hormonal illness can become progressive and even incurable. But take heart. I have found various treatments which are known to decrease symptoms and connect you with all those issues that will need addressing. The irony of this perpetual state of ill health and subsequent depression is that one often feeds off the other, so the cycle of mind–body despair can continue relentlessly into the menopausal years if it isn't treated.

Identifying the triggers for your individual illness is imperative in managing it successfully. For example, if you know that you are approaching your danger time, such as in the luteal phase of your cycle, you will realize the importance of controlling your stress levels (as difficult as that sounds). You will need to stabilize your blood sugar and watch your alcohol consumption, and you will also need to find an exercise regime that will help you to manage your mood swings (with no excuses made). If you are filling in a menstrual chart or using a menstrual app then you will easily be able to identify your cycle and the triggers that exacerbate your condition.

The good news is that things are slowly improving for anyone with problems connected with menstruation. There are now lots of online support networks and forums that can put you in touch with fellow sufferers. These are vital in protecting you from the isolation and loneliness that this misunderstood condition can bring. Unfortunately, in the past there has also been a lack of serious structured protocol for dealing with reproductive depression, but happily that does seem to be changing. In the UK, for instance, the National Institute for Health and Care Excellence (NICE) has issued guidelines that inform all health care practitioners of the correct treatments and standard procedures.

If you are going to see a doctor, or any other health care professional, about your own problems during the luteal phase of your cycle, make sure that you take at least three months' worth of menstrual charts with you (either paper charts or on an app). I also suggest printing off the NICE guidelines for PMS and taking them with you too. This is really important for two reasons. The first is that it shows you have researched and understand your own condition, and the second is that once your health care professional realizes that what you are saying is true, they can follow the valid treatment protocol which is governed by NICE.

Useful websites

NICE guidelines for PMS at https://www.nice.org.uk/guidance
National Association for Premenstrual Syndromes at https://www.pms.org.uk/support/menstrual-diary/

Treatment guidelines for PMS

Nick Panay BSc MRCOG MFSRH

Chairman of the National Association for Premenstrual Syndrome, Director of West London Menopause & PMS Centre, Consultant Gynaecologist Imperial College Healthcare NHS Trust & Chelsea and Westminster NHS Foundation Trust, Honorary Senior Lecturer, Imperial College London

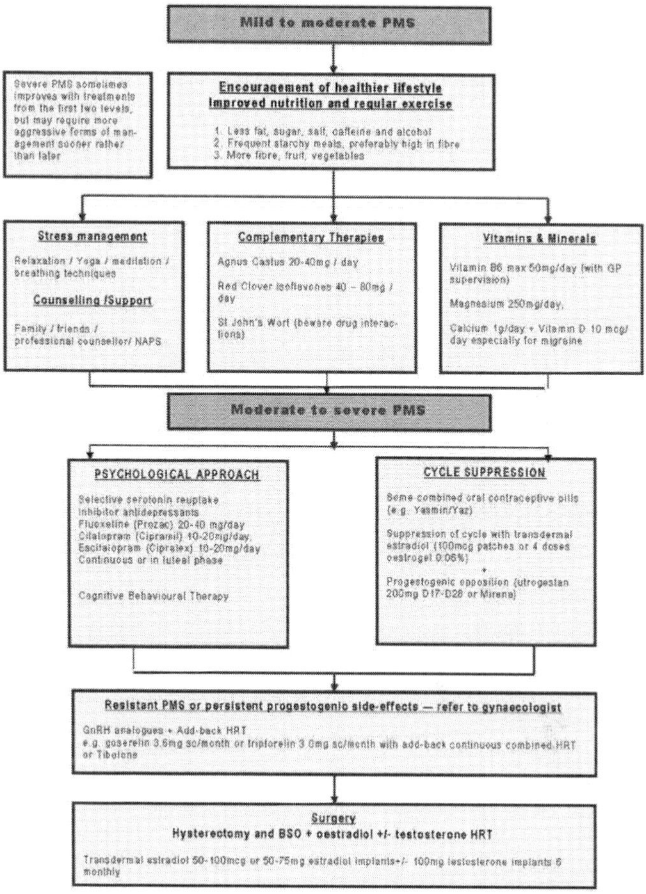

TREATMENTS

There is no single treatment for reproductive depression. We are all different and we all have our own way of coping with our illness. Some prefer to rely on a scientific healing, while others want to maintain a holistic or natural approach, and there is no right or wrong way. However, in my experience, once you have accepted that you are ill and have a biochemical abnormality, you will find your own ways of dealing with this long-term condition. In order to do that, it is essential that you do everything you can to minimize the symptoms. This takes work. It involves re-evaluating every aspect of your life, including mentally, physically and environmentally, so you can gain control over what can be a progressive and indeed a life-threatening illness. You can, of course, use a multi-dimensional approach, which is favoured by most of the people I've come into contact with.

Here are my recommendations of the areas it is worth exploring.

Hormonal Intervention

Ask your doctor for a referral to the nearest gynaecologist or endocrinologist who has the expertise to treat your illness. Do not take no for an answer because you can't do this alone. Make sure that you take with you a menstrual chart, either completed by hand or as an app, or your diary, so you can provide evidence of your changes of mood each month. Ideally, you should take at least three months' worth of charts or diary entries. By the time you have an appointment with the consultant, you will probably have more charts to take with you.

The consultant will probably prescribe one or more hormones which are bioidentical, meaning that at a molecular level they are identical to the hormones your body produces. They aren't the same as pharmaceutical hormones. You might be offered oestrogen, progesterone and sometimes testosterone, in the form of a cream, patch, tablet or even a suppository. You should also be offered blood tests and various scans to see if there are any other abnormalities that are causing your symptoms. You may even be offered a bone scan.

You are usually given a slow and steady dose of the necessary hormones, to avoid your body experiencing the fluctuations which you are so sensitive to. This will stop you having those peaks and troughs which are causing you so many problems. Equally, if you have a baby you will need to avoid the sudden plummet in hormones which often leads to post-natal depression or even a psychotic episode. If your symptoms are very severe, you may be offered an injection to suppress your hormonal system in its entirety. The injection contains a gonadotrophin-releasing hormone antagonist (GnRH) that suppresses the hormones which are causing the problem, and it can even be used to prepare you for a hysterectomy. Once you've had this intervention you should, in theory, have little or no cycle at all and therefore no symptoms. However, the effects of this procedure seem to differ from person to person and there can sometimes be adverse side effects, including a worsening of symptoms.

The last resort, and therefore the most radical option, is the removal of your womb, ovaries and fallopian tubes in the procedure known as BSO. You are normally only offered these procedures if you are suicidal, have underlying disease pathology or, as in my case, both. This surgery can mean an end to the illness, but you may still need to take bioidentical hormones to protect your heart and bones. This is known as 'add-back therapy' and again gives you what you need in a controlled and steady dose, rather than having to live with the fluctuating and destabilizing effects of your own hormones. Together, a hysterectomy and oophorectomy have the ability to transform your life because they can give you a permanent cure.

Even if you do have a hysterectomy and oophorectomy, you will still need to maintain your hormonal equilibrium on a daily basis for the rest of your life. If you don't, you will get poorly and have more physical issues such as brittle bones and a rapid descent into ageing and its associated problems. This is because you will no doubt experience a 'surgical menopause' (one that is induced for medical reasons) which is far more rapid if you don't replace the hormones that are no longer being provided by your ovaries. Once you have had the operation you are simply without your hormone sensitivity which has dominated your life and, indeed, your health.

Be careful, however, of the climacteric phase of the illness, even if you have had a hysterectomy. This is the last stage in your menstrual trajectory and can often be the most troublesome. If you do have problems in this last phase, despite having had a hysterectomy, keep an eye on both your oestrogen and testosterone levels. This is because hormones given transdermally (through your skin, such as a cream or patch) sometimes aren't absorbed as efficiently as, say, the implant. Despite my knowledge of hormonal intervention, I had a really serious episode of depression simply because I wasn't absorbing enough oestrogen from the patch I was wearing.

Wearing the patch lulled me into a false sense of security until I realized what was happening. I had overlooked my declining oestrogen levels and suffered another crisis which, believe it or not, is very common in the climacteric or menopausal phase of this illness. I was then given the implant, both with testosterone and oestrogen which is more easily metabolized when implanted into muscle. Don't be caught out like I was – keep a constant vigil with regards to your overall health. There is absolutely no room for complacency with reproductive depression and you may still need long-term management, even if your uterus has been removed.

Psychiatric Intervention

Even though this illness is clearly hormonal in origin, you may still be prescribed psychiatric medication. This can be extremely helpful, particularly if you have just had a baby, if there is psychosis or if you are suicidal. However, it is my personal opinion that you should always have access to a GP who will organise a referral to the psychiatrist and mental health team who can fully assess the situation and explain the medication and possible side effects. Ask your doctor for a referral. Also, there are a number of mental health crisis centres where you can drop in and find urgent assistance.

If you are in crisis you may be offered a sedative or tranquilizer as a short-term remedy, which can be enormously helpful if you are unable to calm down and sleep. These types of medication are often given in an emergency and in especially if you've just had a baby and are adjusting to the resulting sleep deprivation. However, this powerful medication should only be used in a crisis because it can be addictive and can have adverse side effects if you take it on a long-term basis.

Antidepressants can be immensely helpful and are often prescribed for hormonal depression, again particularly after childbirth. Unfortunately, the newer selective serotonin reuptake inhibitors (SSRIs) can take some time to work, and in the interim the side effects can include nausea, drowsiness, dry mouth and nervousness. However, sometimes it is simply a matter of finding the medication that is most suitable for you, and that can take a while as your body gets used to the effects of the drug. You might find you only need to take antidepressants at ovulation and then for the next two weeks, to help counteract the effects of PMS and PMDD, or you might take them on a more regular basis with amazing results.

Antipsychotics and mood stabilizers are mostly prescribed for a psychotic episode and especially if it happens after the birth of a child. It is my understanding that at this most critical time someone needing this treatment should have access to a community psychiatric nurse and a consultant psychiatrist. They may need to be hospitalized or even sectioned until the situation has resolved, which invariably it does. Both antidepressants and antipsychotics can be used to stabilize the situation, which should always be treated as an emergency. Often getting the patient well again will take some time and their condition must be carefully evaluated by skilled medical professionals in order to protect the life of the patient and, indeed, their child.

There are numerous crisis centres worldwide for anyone in severe emotional distress. Some you can visit in person to be evaluated and others are helplines such as Samaritans, which in 1953 was the first such crisis line to be established in the United Kingdom.

Useful websites

Samaritans at https://www.samaritans.org
SANEline at http://www.sane.org.uk
Mind at https://www.mind.org.uk

Nutrition

If you have hormonal issues there is a possibility that you will have low blood sugar (hypoglycaemia) too, and will sometimes have trouble maintaining your insulin levels. This is a direct result of your endocrine imbalance and is made worse by poor nutrition, hunger and dehydration. This means it's vital that you eat decent food on a regular basis.

Many of us think we are eating good food but are then surprised to discover that we are lacking certain nutrients. Working with a nutritional expert can tell you which nutrients you are deficient in and will help you to eradicate any foods that don't suit you. It is also very likely that you will be lacking some vitamins and minerals, so you must either add them to your diet by eating foods that are rich in them, or take good-quality supplements. Ensuring that you have a good supply of vitamins A, B_6, D and E, as well as zinc, magnesium, chromium and calcium, has been shown to be very beneficial for hormonal illness, and a high-quality essential fatty acid (EFA) will help your body to repair itself.

Menstrual difficulties such as very heavy periods, whether or not they are accompanied by flooding, can lead to anaemia, which is a deficiency in red blood cells. These blood cells carry oxygen round your body, but if you're anaemic they can't carry as much oxygen as normal. This can leave you feeling very tired and lacking in stamina. If it's untreated, anaemia can lead to chronic fatigue, which is a known symptom of hormonal distress. To combat this, you must increase your body's store of iron. Iron supplements in the form of tablets can cause constipation in some people, so a liquid source of iron may suit you better. You also need to increase your daily intake of vitamins B_{12} and D.

As well as knowing what to add to your diet, you need to know what to avoid. It is very common for someone with hormonal disease to have food intolerances as well, and these can worsen during ovulation. Although it may seem illogical, quite often our body craves the very things it doesn't need and may even crave the foods that create an intolerance. These food intolerances cause chronic long-term inflammation which puts even more stress on the system. The most common intolerances involve wheat, dairy, eggs, sugar and yeast, and they often create a digestive imbalance which damages the body even further. The subsequent lowered immunity and decreased mineral absorption creates further toxicity. As I have already explained, intolerance of a certain food means that it doesn't suit you. It's not to be confused with a food allergy, which is when a certain food will do you real harm.

Ideally, you should steer clear of all foods and drinks that cause a spike in your blood sugar, because that will lead to more mood swings and create further problems for your insulin levels. Do your very best to cut out all refined foods and eat the wholemeal or wholewheat equivalents. For instance, ditch white pasta and eat wholewheat or spelt pasta instead, and choose wholemeal, spelt or rye bread (if you can tolerate the wheat and yeast it contains) instead of the white variety. Ideally, if you've got the time you should make your own bread because then you know exactly what goes into it. You must also reduce as much as possible the amount of processed food you eat, especially if the list of ingredients can only be understood by someone with a degree in chemistry. Make sure you have a good supply of fruit and vegetables (fresh or frozen), too, as well as pulses, seeds and nuts if you aren't allergic to them.

When you switch from eating mostly processed and/or refined foods to whole foods, you may find that it takes a while for your digestion to adjust. Make sure that you drink plenty of fresh water every day, as this will help to avoid constipation and/or bloating, which can sometimes happen if you introduce too many fibre-rich foods into your diet at once.

On the subject of what to drink, as I've already explained you must avoid anything that will make your blood sugar levels rise too quickly. This means no sugary drinks, caffeinated drinks including tea and coffee, no chocolate-based drinks and, of course, no alcohol. Alcohol is a particular problem because, as well as depressing your mood in the long term (even if it perks you up at first), it often contains a lot of sugar or is drunk with sugary mixers. It will also sap your willpower, making it more difficult to resist eating those foods you know you should be avoiding.

You may find it very helpful to follow the three-hourly starch diet, developed by Dr Katharina Dalton, which involves eating a starchy snack every three hours with some lean protein to maintain steady blood sugar levels. For instance, I used to eat organic oat cakes and peanut butter. This is extremely effective because it will help to stabilize your mood swings and subsequent irritability. It can also maintain energy levels and give you the restful sleep which is often elusive when you have hormonal problems. The three-hourly starch diet will help to reduce those cravings and balance your hormones. This in turn will increase your serotonin levels and the neurotransmitters which regulate your brain chemistry, and help to combat the effects of stress on your body.

Once you have accepted that your nutritional choices can help with your hormonal cure, it should take around three weeks of intervention to see a difference. Don't expect this to happen overnight! It takes time, acceptance and an abundance of patience to change your hormonal profile, but often the smallest changes can help enormously in bringing about some balance to your system. Many people who I have talked to have seen great positive results simply by changing what they eat, and in particular when they eat it, with the three-hourly starch diet being very helpful. When you're in the late luteal phase of your cycle (in other words, after ovulation), you will need to keep a snack with you at all times to help counteract your mood swings. Sometimes if you wake during the night you may need to eat a starchy snack, and this is vitally important if you have a baby to feed, regardless of whether you are breast-feeding. Eating nutritionally dense food which is unprocessed will be very helpful in combating hormonal problems.

Another element to nutrition is what is now called the microbiome – the microflora that live within our gut. They are essential to our health but they are often out of balance, and that imbalance has been linked to a host of inflammatory and auto-immune conditions. Interest has also been growing with regard to neuro-psychiatric conditions and hormonal disturbances. Healing the gut brain (our guts contain neurotransmitters, as do our brains) and restoring gut health can improve the way we manage emotions and deal with stress. Candida and parasites can lead to irritability and depression, as can food allergies. Maintaining a healthy gut is essential for good overall health and even helps with the absorption of nutritious foods. Taking a decent probiotic can improve your gut microbiome and your brain function, among other things, so look for reputable and high-quality brands such as Udo's Choice and OptiBac in your local independent health food shop. In recent years there has been a lot of publicity about the benefits of fermented foods, because they enhance the role of your gut and also provide extra minerals and antioxidants. Kefir, miso and kombucha are amazing at nourishing the gut and should be eaten every single day.

Counselling and Psychotherapy

Without a doubt, counselling and psychotherapy are immensely powerful when dealing with any form of depression or anxiety, regardless of its cause. These 'talking cures' can help you come to terms with what is happening to you and the fact that you are ill. In my opinion, once you have been diagnosed with a mood disorder you should be under the care of a mental health team who can provide talking therapies and also access to a crisis phoneline. As soon as you are diagnosed you should ask for the input of a Community Psychiatric Nurse who can assess you and establish a care plan, which will give you the support you need.

Cognitive Behavioural Therapy (CBT) is a highly beneficial technique which is immensely helpful at enabling you to conquer negative thoughts and change them into positive and helpful ones. You must be taught by a skilled therapist and you must accept that it's a skill that takes time to master (I took ten weeks) and is often painful and tiring while you learn to restructure your way of thinking. This type of mindfulness can also naturally slow down your thinking, heart rate and breathing, and so then it becomes a kind of meditation. With practice and perseverance, CBT can radically transform your outlook and even improve your hormonal health and immunity. It gives you a chance to delve deeper into childhood trauma or any other underlying issues which may be creating a cycle of stress. Because we now know that stress worsens hormonal problems, it can only help to talk to someone about your illness and its manifestations. Your doctor, or indeed any medical professional, should be able to tell you how to organize some CBT and some will even arrange it for you.

Various forms of counselling may be offered to you, and might include CBT, Dialetical Behavioural Therapy (DBT), regression or Family Constellation Theory. In addition, a decent psychotherapist can often help you come to terms with your condition, particularly if your illness has been severe and you've been having suicidal thoughts. If you don't have access to the professionals then it is vitally important that you can talk to a non-judgemental friend, and preferably one who has the same condition as you. Peer support is absolutely vital and can even save lives, as the person with the illness feels validated and supported by people who understand what they are going through. Online support groups are available on various social media platforms, including Facebook and Twitter.

The IAPMD (International Association of Premenstrual Disorders) has a peer support line where you can talk to someone urgently.

Personally, I try to steer clear of talking to people who don't have emotional issues in case they patronize and undermine me. In my experience it is best to look for support from those who have the illness themselves, or who at least have personal experience of it through a family member or friend. So many times I've tried to explain it to people who either think that I am exaggerating my difficulties or whose dismissive reaction makes me feel ashamed and invalidated.

Another powerful approach is to join a church or fellowship group. I did this myself and found it immensely helpful. The support and spiritual nourishment I received were profoundly and unquestionably beneficial in managing my illness. Once I had accepted that this illness was part of God's plan for me, I was able to connect with Him in a new and appreciative way. This allowed me to come to terms with my trauma and pray about it clearly and concisely, which calmed me and filled me with a sense of peace. I'm perfectly sure that I wouldn't be here if it wasn't for the help and intervention of my Christian friends, their prayers and their belief that one day I would recover. It is recognized that being around spiritual people leads to a sense of peace and tranquillity, particularly when coping with a chronic illness. Spiritual nourishment can quite literally be a spiritual lifeline, and I believe this can be life-saving. It certainly was for me, as I knew that there were people who truly cared about me, were non-judgemental and full of compassion.

Whether you join a church, a meditation circle or even visit the numerous retreats that are available, leading a spiritual life can be life-changing and is often vital in helping you to practise acceptance of your condition. Creating an atmosphere of calm, and grounding yourself in the present, is absolutely essential in the management of emotional illness and can often spell the difference between life and death.

Useful websites

The Integrated Medical Practice at www.drmarkatkinson.com
British Association for Behavioural and Cognitive Psychotherapists (BABCP) at https://www.babcp.com
British Association for Counselling and Psychotherapy (BACP) at https://www.bacp.co.uk
British Psychological Society (BPS) at https://www.bps.org.uk
Counselling and Psychotherapy in Scotland (COSCA) at https://www.cosca.org.uk
UK Association of Humanistic Psychology Practitioners (UKAHPP) at https://ahpp.org.uk
UK Council for Psychotherapy (UKCP) at https://www.psychotherapy.org.uk

Exercise

While writing this part of the book I asked one of the many groups that I am involved in what has helped them most in the management of symptoms and their severity. The answer was exercise. As well as its obvious health benefits, exercise helps to improve lowered immunity and insulin resistance, and it releases endorphins which help to counteract low mood and irritability. It also helps to stabilize all known physical functions and maintains the health of our bones and heart – two areas that can often be compromised by our hormones. Sometimes being unwell will mean that you are unable to do any vigorous exercise, so please bear in mind that even a gentle walk can help enormously, particularly if you're surrounded by nature which itself can be very healing.

If you are suffering from exhaustion as a result of a chattering mind, yoga and/or breath work are among the most calming and grounding exercises that you can do. Some yogic poses are even credited with maintaining pelvic blood flow and regulating hormones. It doesn't need to be high-intensity yoga, provided that you are centred and focused in what you are doing.

Something else you might like to explore is qigong, which works with the body's life force (the 'qi'), using a combination of deep breathing and smooth, flowing movements. Some people describe it as meditation through movement. Some movements will relax you and others will energize you. Medical qigong takes things one step further because it focuses on healing specific physical and mental conditions, including hormonal imbalances. In China, where qigong originated, hospital patients are often healed by practising medical qigong. Tai chi is similar to qigong and consists of flowing sequences of movements. You'll find hundreds of qigong and tai chi videos online, or you could look for a local teacher.

Personally, I enjoy running and other aggressive exercises as they helped me cope with the irritability and the internal rage that consumed me every month during the late luteal phase of my cycle. Vigorous exercise also helps to counter adrenalin overload by reducing the levels of cortisol in the bloodstream. Interval training, in which you slow down and then speed up at intervals, seems to be the most effective exercise for weight management. High-intensity interval training (HIIT), in which you alternate bouts of intense exercise with recovery periods, helps to reduce water retention and premenstrual swelling. Weight-lifting also protects our bones and encourages flexibility and suppleness, all of which can ward off osteoporosis and degeneration of the spine.

All exercise can be used to maintain hormonal health and is absolutely vital when you are trying to minimize your symptoms. Whatever you do, whether it is swimming, walking or something very energetic, make sure that you do it regularly, so that it becomes part of your daily or weekly routine. This helps you to take total charge of your health. If you don't do this, your symptoms can eventually become chronic. So it is really important that we all understand that we need a long-term exercise routine which will lower our stress levels, release those endorphins and balance our endocrine system.

Holistic Approaches

Never before have so many wonderful holistic treatments been available for people with hormonal depression. Most of us will try at least two holistic approaches, if not more, in the long-term aim of keeping our moods on an even keel. Anything that can help us to relax is obviously beneficial, so some people will use a holistic discipline every now and then, while others believe that a holistic approach should be used on a long-term basis because of its health benefits. It is important that you find the approach that works best for you, because we are all different and what appeals to one person may not be right for someone else. So keep an open mind and be prepared to experiment.

Reflexology, in which a trained reflexologist exerts extremely precise pressure on your feet or hands, can be really useful both physically and emotionally. The feet and hands contain a multitude of energy channels (known as meridians) which, once stimulated, have a positive effect on regulating our health. If you've never had reflexology before, don't be surprised if you feel really tired after your first session. That's because the reflexologist will have cleared a lot of toxins and stagnant energy from your body, and you need to give yourself time to recover by resting and also drinking plenty of water to clear your system.

Acupuncture, in which an acupuncturist inserts tiny needles along specific meridians along your body, is also extremely effective, especially for aches and pains and menstrual cramping. Both acupuncture and reflexology can stimulate the body's hormonal pathways to produce more serotonin, so they are always worth a try.

All types of massage are known to release tension and calm the nervous system, with Indian head massage being particularly good for slowing down a chattering mind and easing severe tension. Combining a massage with aromatherapy can stimulate all of your senses, helping to reduce insomnia and tension. Some of the most relaxing aromatherapy oils include lavender, which can help you to sleep, and jasmine, which can not only lull you into a restful sleep but can also reduce anxiety. If you don't want to have an aromatherapy massage you could try adding a few drops of your chosen aromatherapy oils and a few drops of a carrier oil, such as sweet almond oil, to your bathwater, or put a few drops of your chosen oil in a room diffuser. If you are pregnant, you must avoid certain oils, including lavender, because they could trigger a miscarriage.

Some people find Bach Flower Remedies extremely helpful because they work at an emotional level. I have often taken the remedy called Cherry Plum (for fear of losing control) when I've been close to hysteria, and always keep a Rescue Remedy spray (which contains five different Bach remedies) in my bag. There are thirty-eight remedies in all, and you can take a combination of up to seven at any one time. Other Bach Flower remedies that you might find helpful include Olive for mental and/or physical exhaustion, Sweet Chestnut for complete despair, White Chestnut for repetitive thoughts and Gorse for loss of hope that you'll ever get better. When they were first developed in the 1930s, Bach Flower remedies were unique but now you can buy many different forms of flower remedies, such as Australian Bush Essences, and also gem remedies.

Another option to consider is homeopathy. Although you can buy a few homeopathic remedies from most health food shops, if you have a hormonal illness you should really be treated by a professional homeopath on a long-term basis. The consultation, which is more like an in-depth conversation and can last for up to an hour, is an important part of the treatment because it gives you the opportunity to discuss your symptoms and to explore your emotions. The homeopath treats you as an individual and your very specific reaction to a hormonal illness, so the remedies you are prescribed might be very different from those given to another patient with the same hormonal illness. The remedies can work at a very deep level, not only physically but also mentally and emotionally, and they don't have side-effects.

Tapping, which is also known as Emotional Freedom Technique (EFT), can be really helpful, too. It's a technique in which you tap various points on your face, chest and hands while reciting a positive affirmation. This process stimulates the meridian points you're tapping while soothing your body's fight or flight response.

Traditional Chinese Medicine (TCM), which is an ancient form of medicine, can help with hormonal illnesses. The practitioner will talk to you, take your pulses (they will listen to several of your body's pulses, not just one as in western medicine), observe you carefully and establish where disharmony lies in your body. They will then treat you in ways that are designed to restore that harmony.

Many other holistic options are available to you. Eye Movement Desensitization and Reprocessing (EMDR) can help you to deal with any form of post-traumatic stress disorder. Eden Energy Medicine, which was started by Donna Eden, is a combination of several different holistic approaches that work with your energy field, restoring its equilibrium and helping you to stabilize your moods.

If you haven't already explored holistic techniques but you'd like to, you will discover a whole host of different approaches. Find one that really appeals to you and then try it for at least three months to see if it suits you. If you feel slightly anxious about other people knowing that you're trying something that isn't orthodox medicine, it's up to you whether you mention it to them, especially if you're worried that they might sneer or make negative comments about it. We are all different, as I've said before, and what makes sense to one person may seem strange to another, but that doesn't make either of them right or wrong.

Given that hormonal illnesses can be brutal and debilitating, often coinciding with our child-rearing years, I suggest that you seek out anything than can even remotely make you feel better. Quite often, a combination of several different disciplines will be most helpful. You will need to be patient and committed before you find which regime works best for you, because you need to give each one time to work, and it's often a case of trial and error or personal preference. In my own case, and from listening to many other people's experiences, I believe that a combination of medical and integrated health approaches works best.

Useful websites

Association of Reflexologists at https://www.aor.org.uk

Australian Bush Flower Essences at https://www.ausflowers.co.uk

Bach Flower Remedies at https://www.bachremedies.com

British Acupuncture Council at https://www.acupuncture.org.uk

Aromatherapy Council at http://www.aromatherapycouncil.co.uk

Society of Homeopaths at https://homeopathy-soh.org/find-a-homeopath/

EFT at https://www.eftandmindfulness.com/articles/emotional-freedom-technique-eft-43

Traditional Chinese Medicine at https://rchm.co.uk/chinese-medicine

Eden Energy Medicine at https://edenenergymedicine.com

EMDr at https://emdrassociation.org.uk/a-unique-and-powerful-therapy/emdr-the-basics/

Herbs and Minerals

The endless list of herbs and minerals always has a place in the management of any disease, and hormonal conditions are no exception. Some people have experienced amazing results from taking herbs and minerals, and others very little, but the one thing to keep in mind is that each herb and supplementation works differently and with varying degrees from person to person. The one thing to be certain of is that you need to take them regularly and consistently for them to be effective, and you also need to be aware that certain pharmaceutical drugs should not be taken in conjunction with certain herbs. If you are treated by a professional herbalist, which you might find much more effective than prescribing them for yourself, they will ask you about the drugs you have been prescribed and will adapt their treatment when necessary.

Before you take any herbal or mineral supplements you should read up on them in detail so you know what you're doing, especially if you are pregnant, using psychiatric medication or taking any form of hormone replacement. This is because certain preparations can enhance or lessen the effects on your system, and sometimes can even be dangerous.

Here are some suggestions.

St John's Wort is the most promising and well known herb, and is a natu ral anti-depressant. You could try taking 300mg daily. However, if you are taking some form of psychiatric medication you must check with your GP or consultant before taking St John's Wort as it may interfere with the action of the prescribed drugs.

Maca root powder can increase libido, improve mood and is highly nutritious. Make it into a tea or put it in a smoothie.

Chromium when taken in a daily dose of 200mg can balance blood sugar levels and help with food cravings.

5HTP is a known mood booster and a natural serotonin enhancer. Try taking 100mg a day.
Black Cohosh can increase your levels of 'happy hormones' if you take 50mg every day.
Agnus Castus can help to increase the levels of natural hormones, particularly progesterone. Take 4mg daily.
Dong Quai is used to promote hormonal balance and can even help with menstrual cramps. Try taking 600mg daily.
Dandelion is a natural diuretic. You can drink the dried leaves as a tea to reduce water retention. Dandelion even breaks down excess hormones which are no longer needed by the body .
Phytoestrogens and **isoflavones** are highly beneficial and should be used in their most natural state. This means eating organic soya beans, soya milk, tofu and soya yoghurt which are all known to help reverse endocrine 'burn-out'.
L-Tyrosine can help maintain thyroid health and the subsequent auto-immune problems of lowered thyroid function.
Probiotics nourish the gut and are especially helpful to women, but choose a good-quality one, preferably from a health food shop.
Fermented foods can have a profound effect on the gut–brain axis. Kefir, miso and kombucha tea should be staples.
Valerian, camomile and passion flower all have a natural calming and sedative effect that is highly effective, particularly when you are agitated and nervous. I have these in the form of teas, and I inhale the fumes before I drink the tea, which is even more calming.

Useful websites
Herbalism at https://nimh.org.uk

Relaxation Techniques

It can be very hard to relax when you feel depressed or anxious because you're so tense, on edge or keyed up. These symptoms can often lead to insomnia and severe emotional distress. We all react differently to stressful situations, so it's up to you to find that one technique which suits and interests you enough to help with your symptoms. It must be something that you enjoy, so you'll want to keep doing it. My own particular remedy is going to the sauna and steam bath, which has the added bonus of balancing my hormones and boosting immunity. It is also deeply relaxing and I always feel better afterwards, even if I feel reluctant to move.

Gentle music and deep-breathing techniques have powerful health benefits because they centre the mind and allow you to be present in the moment, rather than caught up in distracting thoughts. Breath work can help to reduce anxiety by teaching you to become conscious of your breathing and intentionally slowing it down. Slow breathing tells your nervous system to relax! I use an app called Insight Timer which has a multitude of meditative exercises combining breath work and different forms of mindfulness. In the late luteal phase of my cycle I would practise yoga, long before it was fashionable, and I still do it now. Yoga can even encourage a period to arrive when it's been congested and delayed.

Some people relax by painting or drawing, or have a hobby that can allow them space to wind down. Whatever you choose to do, it's absolutely crucial that you get that sense of tranquillity and peace at least once a week. Building this time into your weekly schedule should be part of a structured self-care plan and is as vital to your health as the food you eat. Make it a habit, just like brushing your teeth. I put aside some time once a day now just for me, and just for me only. This non-negotiable tool (normally exercise, for me) helps with my mental clarity and any overwhelming emotions I'm experiencing.

I know that motivation can be a serious problem for us all, especially when we have such busy lives that finding time for ourselves feels more like an indulgence than a necessity, but you must discover that one thing that helps you, regardless of all of life's challenges and time constraints.

While writing this chapter I asked my peers for their suggestions. It seems that within three months of any restoration programme you'll begin to see some improvement in the intensity of your symptoms and their degree of severity. Allow yourself that three months of self-care for any regime to see if it helps you. If it doesn't, try something else, and keep experimenting until you find what works for you.

Useful websites

Insight Timer at https://insighttimer.com/insighttimer

Know Your Tribe

Knowing your tribe is by far the most important and vital element of your recovery. You will undoubtedly come into contact with people who either don't understand what it means to be in mental crisis or who think that you're pretending, trying to get other people's sympathy or are over-dramatizing the seriousness of your condition. I find this almost as bad as being poorly in itself. One would never argue about their condition with, say, someone with epilepsy or diabetes, yet throughout my entire reproductive years I have found the need to justify my condition and the concept of being unwell.

It seems that unless a person has experienced hormonal disease at first hand, they are reluctant to accept that it can make someone extremely unwell. This is why I've found my tribe, and by that I mean that I refuse to allow myself to be patronized by anyone who doesn't understand the concept of reproductive depression. I no longer try to convince people that I am, or have been, poorly and I refuse to be gaslighted by people who think that someone with a hormonal illness is over-reacting.

Every time someone tries to share their toxic positivity, I turn to someone who does understand and I urge you to do the same. By 'toxic positivity' I mean being told to think positive thoughts, look on the bright side or think of people who are worse off than me, or other similar suggestions. I found my tribe mostly online in support groups and it's been invaluable in my recovery and acceptance of this condition. People who are unsupportive can be very triggering, which in turn can harm our thought processes and even intensify an episode. You know the truth. You know you are unwell, so don't let other people tell you otherwise. Don't let other people undermine the severity of your condition. Having a hormonal disease is very serious and it must be acknowledged.

Finding your tribe can be as important as finding the correct doctor, researching the latest treatments and eating nutritious foods. All of us who connect swap ideas and treatment protocols, and many lives have been saved as a result. I wouldn't have found out about Professor Studd's work if I hadn't reached out to others with hormonal depression and I also wouldn't have been able to write this testimony, which will undoubtedly validate the experiences of many others with this illness.

Look for supportive, understanding and compassionate people who can surround you with love. They will know that you cannot simply make your illness go away through sheer willpower, so being in touch with them could be the most important element of your recovery. It could even save your life.

Useful websites

Peer Support Team for IAPMD at https://iapmd.org/peer-support-team

EXTRA HELP AND SUPPORT

Here are some additional ideas, techniques and suggestions.

Educate Yourself

The most valuable piece of advice I could give to any sufferer is to educate yourself in every possible way, and with every available source that you can find. The more you know about this illness and all of its manifestations, the better. Believe me, there is lots to know and a huge amount of ongoing research within universities across the world and with various health organizations.

Judging by recorded history, we are living in a privileged era because in previous centuries the methods for treating hormonal illnesses were often barbaric and extreme. In the nineteenth century women with hormonal conditions were regarded as hysterical lunatics and sometimes endured the removal of ovaries, often without anaesthesia or any other kind of pain relief. The condition was recognized very early in historical documentation and it was noted that the late luteal phase of a woman's cycle could often give rise to 'moments of temporary insanity which could be attributed to masturbation or far too much reading and singing'. Although this is both ill-informed and possibly laughable, it does confirm that this condition isn't new. In the late nineteenth century it was noticed that mental asylums housed far more women than men.

Fortunately there are now societies, associations and numerous publications which can help someone to decide if their condition is caused by their hormones, and this can be extremely empowering and often life-changing. With the help of the best specialists and the most up-to-date research, you can decide on the best course of action and then the best hormonal therapy for your individual needs. Quite often it is a case of trial and error until the most successful combination of hormones can be found, but this involves a long-term strategy if it's going to be effective.

Ten Things You Can Do To Help Yourself

Since I started practising acceptance, things have become slightly more bearable in terms of managing my symptoms and knowing what's around the corner. I believe that this is because I have time to prepare and I am much more aware of my triggers. Getting enough sleep, for example, is a priority for me, but so is sticking to the same sleep pattern because that teaches my brain when it's time for me to go to sleep and when it's time to wake up. All organisms have this circadian rhythm, but for us it is very closely linked with the menstrual cycle, and therefore a disturbed circadian rhythm will contribute to a disturbed menstrual cycle. It is also important to manage any highly stressful situations.

You must try to become aware of what's going on in your body throughout each month. For example, there is little point in pretending that you can't feel something brewing when you know that you have just ovulated and that this is the most difficult phase in your cycle. It is futile to try to overcome hormonal depression in the days leading up to your period and likewise you should accept that you may have problems after childbirth and also during menopause. In other words, as part of your self-care programme, you must plan ahead.

When writing this chapter I asked members of the many groups to which I belong what they do to help them cope. The list below is. Here are ten strategies, which are a combination of my ideas and their suggestions, that could make all the difference to your life each month.

- Follow the three-hourly starch diet by eating a starchy snack every three hours on the dot. Eat within one hour of waking and one hour before sleep. Try to only eat nutritious foods throughout your cycle, and at the very least during the late luteal phase of your cycle each month. Clean up your diet and stick to this new regime because it will help to reduce adrenalin and cortisol overload.
- Follow a meticulous exercise routine every day, regardless of how tired or short of time you are. You must prioritize this even if it's only a ten-minute walk. Increase the time daily, using one of the many exercise apps which are available, and you will be amazed at how quickly you can reduce your symptoms.
- Buy an anxiety blanket. Whenever you feel overwhelmed or out of control, take yourself away from the situation you are in and lie under the blanket. It gives you a cuddle, quite literally, and can help with the mental chatter and also misophonia that you may be experiencing.
- Make sure you prioritize your sleep and try to go to sleep at the same time every night. This helps to 'balance' the menstrual clock in your brain and even out your fluctuating hormones. Tiredness is an enemy because it exacerbates depression and anxiety, so make sure you are getting adequate rest. If you are tired you tend to eat more sugary foods to give yourself a boost, and that will lead to peaks and subsequent troughs in your insulin levels, which will make you feel even more tired.
- Do not drink alcohol, at least in the late luteal phase. Ideally, giving up totally should be the ultimate aim for anyone with a hormonal illness. Unfortunately, self-medicating with

alcohol helps at the time but there will be a period of 'hangxiety' (a combination of hangover and anxiety) afterwards, and even a deep depression. Stay away from wine especially, as it is mostly sugar and therefore interferes with the metabolism of your hormones. It also causes dehydration, which means that your body cannot function correctly. If you really must have a drink, clear spirits are best because they contain fewer sulphites than wine. If necessary, add a non-sugary mixer.

- Join some of the many various online forums and get a support network around you. There are literally hundreds to choose from, ranging from those dealing with teenage problems to the menopausal transition. Being a member of these forums can help you to combat the feelings of isolation and loneliness that often accompany any emotional issues. Make friends with people who have the same disorder and stay connected. You will be helping them and they will be helping you.
- Meditation and relaxation techniques should be an important part of your routine. Be patient when searching for something that suits you because sometimes it can take a while to find a technique that you really like. Whether you choose yoga, deep-breathing techniques, qigong or something else, keep practising and eventually it will become second nature. There is a saying that it takes twenty-one days for something to become a habit, so give it a good three weeks to work. Look for any suitable groups that are local to you or, if you don't feel like mixing with people, look for an online group that appeals to you.
- Find a decent health care provider and ask them to help you produce a new care plan. If this doesn't work or if your doctor is unhelpful, as is often the case, keep looking until you find a doctor who will help you. Don't be discouraged by dismissive comments, and make sure you take evidence of your

condition with you in the form of your menstrual chart or the details from your app. Print off the NICE guidelines and insist that your doctor follows them to the letter. This alone can be very empowering. Help is available and you should have access to it.

- Eco-therapy and spending time in nature is a marvellous form of medicine. Getting out into a green environment such as a park or a forest is vital for both your physical and mental well-being. It also has the added bonus of providing extra sunlight (weather permitting, of course), and that can induce a sense of quiet calmness. This reduces both stress and anger and can even improve your confidence. Find that space and go there whenever necessary. A private place in nature can be your own little sanctuary. If you can't face travelling far, or it isn't possible, you could create a little retreat space in your own garden if you have one. Alternatively, if you really can't get out but you'd love to, visit your favourite space in your imagination or look at photos you've taken of it. Make this as vivid an experience as possible. Use visualisation techniques, and keep practising.
- Keep the number of your nearest crisis centre to hand. If you are despairing, please make that call. There is always someone at the end of that phoneline and asking for help is vital if you are in crisis. You have no need to feel ashamed or worried about people's perceptions of you. Most people who work in crisis centres or on helplines have overcome huge obstacles themselves, and they will have been trained so they know how to respond in a constructive and compassionate way. Remember that tomorrow is another day. Write this down where you can see it, to give yourself strength, and look at it every day.

Outside Support

To me, by far the most important association in the world is the International Association for Premenstrual Disorders (IAPMD). It was founded as the National Association for Premenstrual Dysphoric Disorder (NAPMDD) by Amanda LaFleur and Sandi MacDonald in 2013 and became the IAPMD in 2018. It is a non-profit organization that aims to inspire hope and end suffering for all those affected by hormonal illnesses. It is a lifeline of support, information and resources and also runs a peer-support programme. It is committed to research and is passionate about raising awareness of hormonal illness. You can also read scientific papers on their website, which has a unique provider directory so you can locate your nearest doctor who can treat PMDD. You will find an immense amount of information on their website at iapmd.org

There are some other excellent associations too. The National Association for Premenstrual Syndromes (NAPS) offers an abundance of information, including the latest therapies, regular bulletins and a list of specialists who can help. You can also donate money and receive details of upcoming events and support. You will find more details on their website at https://www.pms.org.uk

The Association for Post Natal Illness (APNI) provides masses of information, has support groups and is passionate about raising awareness of post-natal depression. They can also advise families and health professionals should the need arise. Their website is at https://apni.org

PMDD & Me CIC provides evidence-based education and support for anyone who has menstrual difficulties. It was founded by Alice Girling and her wife Sarah, and in 2019 organized the first UK conference for people who are affected by PMDD. A former midwife, Alice is passionate about raising awareness, and is committed to sharing resources and educating health care providers. She also hosts various webinars and podcasts with other senior health care professionals. The PMDD and Me CIC website is at https://pmddandme.co.uk

Samaritans is a UK-based crisis service that can be contacted on 08457 90 90 90. They are available twenty-four hours a day, seven days a week, for anyone who needs them, whether they are a sufferer of hormonal disease or otherwise, and have saved many lives in doing so. Their website is at https://www.samaritans.org

Dr Katharina Dalton is the author of *Depression after Childbirth: How to Recognize, Treat and Prevent Postnatal Depression*, now a classic text, which gives a perfect explanation of post-natal depression and how it can be managed by hormonal intervention. Dr Dalton also wrote *The PMS Bible*, once again advocating the use of hormonal therapies and dietary needs (including the three-hourly starch diet) during the week leading up to menstruation.

Dr Patrick Holford has published many books and has a special interest in hormones and nutrition. His books *Balance Your Hormones* and *The Feel Good Factor* are both extremely useful on how to manage all aspects of health and medicine, both natural and otherwise. His website is at https://www.patrickholford.com

Dr Mark Atkinson, author of *The Mind Body Bible*, combines conventional medicine with natural and bioidentical supplementations and also has clinics and workshops across the UK. You can contact him at https://www.drmarkatkinson.com

Professor John Studd, who is a consultant gynaecologist in Harley Street, London, can be contacted at E.harley@studd.co.uk He also has an amazing website which should be a first call for any sufferer, if only to read the latest research and findings, at https://www.studd.co.uk/index.php As far as knowledge and expertise go, Professor Studd is the leading practitioner on hormonal illness.

Claire Louise Knox has founded See her Thrive, which is dedicated to ensuring that women's health is understood and supported in the workplace. She has an amazing website at www.seeherthrive.com

Laura Murphy is co-founder of Vicious Cycle which is passionate about raising awareness and making PMDD visible. She is also committed to raising the standards of care for those with menstrual disorders. Laura's website is at https://www.viciouscyclepmdd.com

Dr Christiane Northrup is an obstetrician and gynaecologist. She has written several books about women's health, including *The Wisdom of Menopause* and the classic *Women's Bodies, Women's Wisdom*. Her website, which is full of valuable information, is at https://www.drnorthrup.com

Memoirs

Here are some memoirs describing some women's experiences of hormonal illness.

Eyes Without Sparkle: A Journey Through Postnatal Illness by Elaine A Hanzack, Routledge, 1998

Out of Me: A Memoir of Postnatal Depression by Fiona Shaw, Penguin, 1998

Laugh in the Face of PMS Diary by Susan Callery, Susan Callery, 2011

The Madwoman in the Volvo: My Year of Raging Hormones by Sandra Tsing Loh, Norton, 2015

Lost Marbles: Insights into My Life with Depression and Bipolar by Natasha Tracy, CreateSpace Independent Publishing Platform, 2016

Whichever route you decide to go down, whether it be conventional or holistic, knowledge is the most powerful weapon you have and should be a continuous strategy in your recovery if it's to be for the long term.

GLOSSARY

Amenorrhoea The absence of menstrual periods.

Bioidentical hormones Hormones which are identical at a molecular level with endogenous hormones.

Climacteric The period of life when fertility and sexual activity are in decline. In women, this is the menopause.

Comorbidity The simultaneous presence of two or more diseases in a patient.

Corpus luteum The remains of the ovarian follicle that has released a mature egg.

Chronic post-traumatic stress disorder (CPTSD) A disorder resulting from repeated trauma over a number of years.

Dopamine An organic hormone and brain transmitter.

Dysmenorrhea Painful and problematic menstrual periods.

Fallopian tube One of a pair of tubes along which the egg travels from the ovary to the uterus.

Follicle-stimulating hormone (FSH) A chemical responsible for the growth of ovarian follicles and which helps to maintain the female menstrual cycle.

Gonadotrophin hormones Hormones which act on the testes and ovaries to stimulate either sperm or ova respectively.

Homeostasis The state of steady, internal, physical and chemical conditions that maintain the body's optimal function.

Hormone A chemical messenger that is secreted directly into the blood and is carried to the relevant organ or tissue in order to fulfil its function.

Hypothalamus A gland in the brain that is responsible for metabolic processes and neuro-endocrine function, and also control of the pituitary gland.

Luteal phase The second half of the menstrual cycle, starting at ovulation and ending on the first day of menstruation.

Luteinising hormone (LH) A hormone produced by the pituitary gland which controls the reproductive system.

Menopause The easing and ending of menstruation to mark the end of the female reproductive years.

Misophonia A neurological condition in which certain sounds trigger negative emotional and physiological responses, and therefore activate the flight or fight response.

Neuro-immune response Alterations in the function of the nervous system which influence the immune response.

Oestrogen A sex hormone responsible for the development and regulation of the female reproductive system and secondary sex characteristics.

Osteoporosis A bone disease that occurs when the body loses too much bone density, makes too little bone, or both.

Ovary The female reproductive organ that produces an ovum.

Ovulation The process by which the ovary releases a mature egg which then moves down the fallopian tube and into the uterus to await fertilization.

Paraben A synthetic chemical used in a wide range of products, including cosmetics and shampoos, to give them a longer shelf life. Their names include butylparaben, isobutylparaben, methylparaben and propylparaben. The structure of parabens is similar to that of oestrogen.

Perimenopause The natural transition into menopause.

Pituitary gland A pea-sized gland at the base of the brain which is important in controlling growth and development and the functioning of other endocrine glands.

Placenta The organ present in the uterus during pregnancy. It provides the growing baby with oxygen and nutrients. It is attached to the wall of the uterus by the umbilical cord.

Post-partum The first six weeks after giving birth.

Premenstrual dysphoric disorder (PMDD) A severe form of premenstrual syndrome.

Premenstrual syndrome (PMS) Adverse symptoms experienced before the menstrual cycle which are cyclical and require treatment.

Premenstrual tension (PMT) Difficult symptoms that occur before the menstrual cycle but are not as severe as those of PMS.

Progesterone A female sex hormone released by the corpus luteum in the ovary. It plays important roles in the menstrual cycle and the early stages of pregnancy.

Progestin A synthetic form of progesterone.

Serotonin A complex neurotransmitter responsible for multiple bodily functions including mood, digestion, sexual function and sleep.

Testosterone A sex hormone which plays a key role in male reproduction but is also present in females.

ACKNOWLEDGEMENTS

To my husband Den who has quite literally saved me.

To my lovely mum who must at times have despaired of me.

To the amazing Jane Struthers for her professional contribution to this book and for her invaluable expertise in both the editing process and healthcare advice.

To my dear friends Samantha Fountain and Lucy Alexander who helped with technical support and glitches.

To Amanda Lafleur and Sandi Macdonald of IAPMD whose tireless work has undoubtedly saved lives.

For my friends Gina, Caroline and my oldest bestie Rubes whose continuous fight and amazing courage is an example to us all.

To Alice Girling who remains 'with women' and always fights their corner.

To Mr Nick Panay of the Chelsea and Westminster Hospital who said the words 'I believe you'.

For my beautiful little boys. I hope I haven't embarrassed you. You were so worth all of it and there are no words to describe how much you are wanted and loved.

And, last but not least, Professor John Studd, whose contribution to helping all women worldwide can never be measured. His professionalism and knowledge have undoubtedly transformed the lives of millions and continue to do so.

Printed in Great Britain
by Amazon

)64306R00092